Dictionary of
Transactional
Analysis

Dictionary of Transactional Analysis

Tony Tilney
Thanet Centre for Psychotherapeutic Studies
Birmingham

Consulting Editor: Professor Windy Dryden
Goldsmiths College, University of London

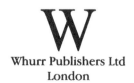
Whurr Publishers Ltd
London

© 1998 Whurr Publishers

First published 1998 by
Whurr Publishers Ltd
19b Compton Terrace, London N1 2UN, England

Reprinted 1999, 2001, 2004, 2005, 2006 and 2007

British Library Cataloguing-in-Publication Data
A catalogue record for this book is available from the British Library.

ISBN-13: 978 1 86156 022 3 p/b

Contents

Acknowledgements

I should like to thank Adrienne Lee for giving me access to previously unpublished material and pre-publication access to her chapter on process in *Contracts in Counselling* (Lee, 1997), Ian Stewart for giving me pre-publication access to his chapter on the history of transactional analysis in *Developments in Psychotherapy, Historical Perspectives* (Stewart, 1996a), Mairi Evans and Andy Fookes for the entry on Gestalt therapy, Andy Fookes for the entry on person-centred therapy, Paul Richards for the entry on NLP and to Ann Smith for her ideas on the 'drowning person' diagram. I am also grateful to Mairi Evans for constructive criticism and helpful advice.

My thanks also go to Chris Davidson who did an outstanding job in creating the diagrams.

I am grateful to the copyright holders for permission to reproduce the following material which forms part of this book.

The Institute of Transactional Analysis, the European Association for Transactional Analysis and the International Transactional Analysis Association for the use of their codes of ethics.

From the Transactional Analysis Journal (TAJ) and the Transactional Analysis Bulletin (TAB).

John Dusay for *the Egogram*: TAJ (1972) 2:3.
Franklin Ernst for *the OK corral*. TAJ (1971) 1:4.
Richard Erskine and Marilyn Zalcman for *the Racket System*: TAJ (1979) 9:1.
Taibi Kahler PhD for *the Miniscript*: TAJ (1974) 4:1.
Stephen Karpman for *the Drama Triangle*: TAB (1968) 7:26.
Ken Mellor for *Impasses: a developmental and structural understanding*: TAJ (1980) 10:3.
Ken Mellor and Eric Sigmund for *the Discount Matrix*: TAJ (1975) 5:3.

Introduction

Understanding what transactional analysis is about

To understand transactional analysis it is essential to know something of its history. Eric Berne, its founder, after qualifying as a psychiatrist, decided to train in psychoanalysis. This approach concentrates on intrapsychic (within the mind) changes and gives little weight to interactions between people.

Psychoanalysis, like many other psychotherapeutic approaches, is essentially a one-person psychology. In his work as a psychiatrist, Berne became increasingly interested in the interpersonal dimension. Harry Stack Sullivan (1953) had started to look at this from a position somewhat outside the mainstream of psychoanalysis. Berne's original objective was to extend psychoanalysis into the interpersonal field and he published a series of papers on this topic in professional journals. As he developed his ideas they met increasing resistance from psychoanalysts. He eventually decided to terminate his training in psychoanalysis and establish a new school, which he called *transactional analysis* (he had already chosen the term *transaction* for the unit of interpersonal interaction). This added the analysis of interpersonal interactions to the analysis of intrapsychic processes and integrated the two viewpoints – people's private experiences and how they behaved towards each other – to create a two-person psychology. He thus brought together the insights of the psychoanalysts with the objectivity of the behaviourists. He developed new theory, in particular concerning *ego-states*, which made this integration possible. He added a third element, his personal philosophical position rooted in humanistic values. He sought to value and empower his patients (a central principle of transactional analysis is that everyone can think and make decisions for themselves) and so set up relations with them that were open, respectful and authentic. To this end he set out to turn theory into a shared resource that can be used by both client and therapist. This involved clarifying, demystifying and finding simple ways of representing key elements.

He set out his theories in a brilliant book *Transactional Analysis in Psychotherapy* (Berne, 1961) which had little immediate impact. He then wrote a book on one aspect of his ideas, *games theory*. *Games People Play* (Berne, 1964) became a worldwide best seller and transactional analysis had a meteoric start unique in psychotherapy. This early success brought both fame and misunderstanding as this book contains only a brief outline of transactional analysis theory. *Games People Play* remains the book by which Berne and transactional analysis are best known but games theory developed rapidly after its publication and much of this book is now seriously out of date.

Using this dictionary

Words printed in capitals indicate that more information can be obtained by looking under that heading in the dictionary. Note that the dictionary entry may not be identical with the capitalised word, as the latter has to conform to the grammatical requirements of the sentence in which it occurs (for example, you will find information on TRANSACTING under transactions).

If you have had little previous contact with transactional analysis you will find it helpful to look first at the following entries:

Berne, Eric
ego-states
transactions
games
script
methodology of transactional analysis
language of transactional analysis
theoretical stance of transactional analysis
philosophy of transactional analysis
history of transactional analysis
message format
schools of transactional analysis
literature of transactional analysis

Dictionaries are usually thought of as providing definitions. A technical dictionary like this also needs to provide explanations. These are not always the same thing. An explanation is designed to build understanding. A definition sets boundaries to the term so that a decision can be made as to what does and what does not fall into the category. A definition does not become meaningful until the explanation has been understood. Sometimes both functions can be held in one process; a clear explanation clarifies boundaries, a good definition conveys the essence of the idea. Sometimes the tasks of explaining and defining have to be addressed separately. I hope I have kept a proper balance between the two.

Transactional analysis presents unique problems in selecting words to include in a dictionary. These problems derive from its unusual history. Transactional analysis grew out of psychoanalysis, in which Eric Berne trained. He and the other founders set out to eliminate any terms that were unessential and to find, wherever possible, specifiable behaviours that could be linked to the terms. There was therefore a major shift in the direction of behavioural definitions; for example, the term *transference* almost disappeared but many behaviour patterns that involved transference were named (such as games, scripts, rackets, drivers, rubberbanding, complementary transactions). The theory thus became less abstract and more accessible and 'user friendly'. At the same time TA expanded in a number of fields: education, organisations, self-help groups, counselling and psychotherapy. Its concrete and straightforward style made it successful in the first three. However, in psychotherapy it sought to establish itself as a depth psychology and increase the range of psychological conditions it was prepared to address. As this occurred it found itself increasingly cramped by the discarding of intrapsychic language. Two approaches were adopted to address this problem: an elaboration of transactional analysis theory to fill the gap and borrowing from psychoanalysis. The latter has become increasingly important, particularly drawing on those areas of psychoanalysis that had expanded or originated after TA split off in the 1960s, namely object relations and self psychology. A significant point was when Carlo Moiso was given the Eric Berne Memorial Scientific Award in 1987 for his article on Ego-states and transference (Moiso, 1985), integrating TA and psychoanalytic concepts. This was followed by an increasing number of articles written from an integrative standpoint (such as Clark, 1991). There was another obvious change: before 1985 TA tended to look inwards and articles were almost exclusively referenced to other TA articles. Now, looking through the *Transactional Analysis Journal*, many of the references are to sources outside TA. Ian Stewart (1996a) has called this process 'the psychoanalytic renaissance'. It has sometimes generated tensions among transactional analysts, some of whom fear that TA may lose its crispness and objectivity if it veers too far towards psychoanalysis, whereas others believe that too close an adherence to past patterns may impede growth. A dictionary of TA must reflect the field as a whole. I have therefore included the major concepts of TA but have also provided resources needed to read a contemporary advanced article by one of the major integrative writers such as Richard Erskine. This involved including a substantial number of non-TA words. The criterion I have used for selecting these words is to include:

- Words used by Eric Berne (who trained as a psychoanalyst) and which are therefore essential to understanding the core literature of TA. An example is *ego-dystonic*.
- Words borrowed by transactional analysts and in widespread use – and therefore essential if the dictionary is to enable a reader to make sense of the current literature e.g. *Gestalt, attachment, holding, containment*.
- Words from other disciplines relating to ideas that have been, or are being, integrated into transactional analysis (e.g. depressive position, projective identification). The non-TA origin of all these words is clearly indicated.

Writing this dictionary focused my attention on how problematic is the function of words in conveying meaning. The setting out of a word suggests that there is a precise meaning that can be conveyed to the reader, but the ultimate source of all meaning is experience (including experience of other meaning structures) and the reader may lack this. As Wilfred Bion, the object relations theorist, pointed out, a function of terminology is to create spaces into which meaning may enter. He wrote: 'the advantage of employing a sign ... is that it at least indicates that the reader's comprehension of my meaning should contain an element that will remain unsatisfied until he meets the appropriate realisation.' For example, a dictionary may contain a definition of the word 'elephant'. However good this is, it can give little idea of what the experience of seeing an elephant would be like. However, the definition is good enough if, after reading it, anyone seeing an elephant for the first time thinks immediately 'that must be an elephant'. It is a tempting for the dictionary-maker to labour overmuch at defining elephants. I hope I have avoided this.

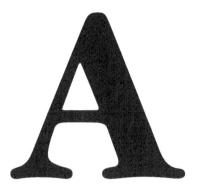

A Layman's Guide to Psychiatry and Psychoanalysis Eric Berne's first book, originally published under the title THE MIND IN ACTION in 1947 and so predating the emergence of transactional analysis as a separate discipline. This looked mainly at classical (DRIVE THEORY) PSYCHOANALYSIS but is enlivened by Berne's lucid, friendly and humorous style. Revised editions incorporating some transactional analysis were published under the title *The Layman's Guide to Psychiatry and Psychoanalysis* in 1957 and 1967, the latter edition also incorporating contributions from other transactional analysts.

abreaction a release of emotion occurring (usually) in the course of therapy or counselling as a result of contacting Child ego-state experiences.

accreditation recognition by a professional organisation. For transactional analysts in the UK this body is the Institute of Transactional Analysis (ITA), which is affiliated to the European Association for Transactional Analysis (EATA). Accredited transactional analysts are known as certified transactional analysts (CTA). Certification may be obtained in different specialities (clinical, organisational, educational, counselling). Certified transactional analysts in the UK may apply for professional membership of the Institute of Transactional Analysis. As the ITA is a member organisation of the United Kingdom Council for Psychotherapy (the major governing body for psychotherapy in the UK), transactional analysts with clinical speciality become UKCP registered psychotherapists. Most national and regional transactional analysis associations are linked by a system of agreements with the International Transactional Analysis Association (ITAA) and as a result there is mutual recognition of qualifications worldwide.

acting out expressing unresolved psychological issues through behaviour. This brings some relief from psychological pain by providing a channel for repressed feelings but maintains the denial so the issues remain unresolved. Acting out often involves the expression of RACKET feelings and is central to GAMES.

activities one of the six modes of TIME STRUCTURING (Berne, 1964) that are used to satisfy STRUCTURE HUNGER, the others being withdrawal, rituals, pastimes, games and intimacy in order of increasing potentialities for stroking and also of increasing risk of rejection. Unlike the other forms of time structuring,

1

activities are primarily directed to the achievement of goals in the here and now. The predominant ego-state tends to be Adult and since the goals are often material rather than social, stroking and social risk are variable.

adaptation adapting to the perceived or fantasised needs of others (initially the parents). See ADAPTED CHILD.

adapted Child (often written Adapted Child) the Child ego-state functioning in response to Parent demands rather than its own needs. It may be compliant or rebellious. The adapted Child does not represent a separate internal (interpsychic) structure but is one of the ways the Child ego-state shows itself in behaviours. This concept is therefore most useful when we are viewing the person mainly from a behavioural perspective, e.g. analysing transactions. See EGO-STATES FUNCTIONAL MODEL and FALSE SELF.

Adult ego-state often written Adult. The ego-state that deals with 'here and now' reality. Some transactional analysis writing offers a somewhat limited and mechanistic model of the Adult, which is compared to a computer. However, any response that is appropriate to current reality is an Adult response and this can include emotions.

adult survivor an adult who suffered sexual, physical or emotional abuse in childhood.

advantages of games (reasons for playing games) see GAMES, ADVANTAGES OF.

advocacy the therapeutic approach in which the therapist becomes the advocate of the Child in the client against his or her persecuting Parent ego-state. The psychoanalyst Alice Miller (1983, 1985) has written extensively about this approach. Also see ALLIANCE.

affect emotion, feeling. Transactional analysis recognises four AUTHENTIC FEELINGS: sadness, anger, happiness ('sad, mad, glad') and fear. Each of these, in the right context, can lead to dealing constructively with life issues (although they can also be expressed inappropriately or manipulatively in a RACKETY way). Other feelings are more complex and include cognitive elements. For example, guilt involves beliefs about moral failure, or shame about shortcomings being known to others.

affirmation a positive statement (often a self-statement) used to raise self-esteem and to reinforce new and more positive ways of thinking, feeling and behaving. Affirmations intervene in the SCRIPT SYSTEM by changing beliefs about self and also by promoting non-scripty fantasies in place of fantasies which supported script.

agenda a list of things to be dealt with. In therapy the client (and sometimes the therapist) may have a hidden agenda of assumptions, intentions and wishes that are not made explicit (and may not even be consciously acknowledged). One of the main functions of CONTRACTING is to make hidden agendas explicit. Contracting is thus not only a prelude to the therapeutic process but is an important therapeutic technique to which one may have to turn repeatedly as therapy proceeds. Transactional analysis therapy is a contractual process and in the process the therapist constantly makes explicit what is being done and invites the client's consent, so in addition to the macro process in which a formal therapy contract is negotiated, contracting is going on at the micro level.

agitation one of the FOUR PASSIVE BEHAVIOURS (Schiff and Schiff, 1971). This is shown by repeated purposeless behaviours. It occurs when there has been a build-up of undischarged tension because of failure to act to have needs met. This is a passive behaviour because the energy is discharged in a way that is not directed to solving the problem. An example would be fidgeting because a lecturer is inaudible instead of directing the energy into asking him to speak up.

alcoholism addiction to, abuse of, alcohol. This is regarded by some as a disease, the view taken by Alcoholics Anonymous. Transactional analysis regards alcoholism and other forms of SUBSTANCE ABUSE as involving the ACTING OUT ('playing GAMES') of underlying psychological problems. These may involve unresolved SYMBIOSIS, an attempt by the person to become looked after as he or she was (or sought to be) as a child. See Steiner (1971). See also CODEPENDENCY.

alliance a therapeutic technique in which the therapist or a projection of some figure from the client's past experience acts as the Child's ally in dealing with a persecuting Parent. This may be done using GUIDED FANTASY in which the client is invited to remember an incident from his or her past and bring in the ally or by CUSHION WORK in which the client is invited to project parts of himself or herself, e.g. the child of a certain age that he or she once was, incorporated or introjected figures ('people they carry inside themselves') on to cushions and become each of them in turn by sitting on the cushion. See also ADVOCACY.

The positive relationship between the client and therapist which is the prerequisite of therapy is known as the THERAPEUTIC ALLIANCE.

allowers these are the opposites ('antidotes') to DRIVER messages (Kahler and Capers, 1974). They are:

Be Perfect	You're good enough as you are
Please Others	Please Yourself
Be Strong	Be open and express your wants
Hurry Up	Take your time
Try Hard	Do it.

Drivers form part of the COUNTERSCRIPT, which is mainly responsible for how people behave while the SCRIPT PROPER holds the major damage in the form of the INJUNCTIONS. Drivers therefore form a very obvious part of people's problems and it might seem that getting rid of the drivers will solve them. However drivers also have a defensive function: they are a way of getting an OK feeling to counter the negative effect of the injunctions. In therapy it is better to leave the drivers in place until there is sufficient PROTECTION to counter the negative effect of injunctions when they are removed. The DROWNING PERSON DIAGRAM illustrates the protective function of drivers. The removal of a driver message by deciding to act differently constitutes the resolution of a type 1 impasse. See REDECISION SCHOOL, IMPASSE.

almost I script a PROCESS SCRIPT (Berne, 1970, 1972) type in which success is almost achieved but is sabotaged at the last moment (e.g. work hard to achieve promotion and then mess up the interview). The almost I script may also be expressed in unfinished projects. The characteristic driver pattern is Please Others + Try Hard.

almost II script a PROCESS SCRIPT (Berne, 1970, 1972) type in which success is achieved but never satisfies, so a higher goal is immediately substituted for the previous one (e.g. decide you want a degree, work hard to get it, decide that a first degree does not count and enrol for a PhD, climb the ladder in a university to a professorship, this also does not satisfy and you set your heart on becoming a Fellow of the Royal Society and so on). The characteristic driver pattern is Please Others + Be Perfect.

always script a PROCESS SCRIPT (Berne, 1970, 1972) type in which the same pattern occurs over and over. People with this script type keep getting into the same type of situation (e.g. relationship failures) and although they may think each time that they understand what went wrong and will not make that mistake again, somehow, in a new set of circumstances, they do. This is characteristically associated with a Try Hard driver.

anal stage (psychoanalysis) in Freudian developmental theory the stage that occurs between the ages of two and four and involves the investment of LIBIDO in the anus. Concern with the control of defecation may form the basis of later control and obsessional problems. The obsessive compulsive and passive aggressive PERSONALITY ADAPTATIONS are established at this stage.

anger an emotion elicited by obstruction to the satisfaction of one's needs and wishes by others and also by threats to the self or aspects of the self (e.g. from a physical attack to a slighting remark). Used appropriately, anger generates an active and assertive approach to solving interpersonal problems and is a useful signal to others. Anger is often repressed as a result of being disallowed by parents. Repressed anger may be redirected against the self and is then the source of many psychological problems, in particular of depression and low self-esteem. Anger is one of the FOUR AUTHENTIC FEELINGS.

anger work a therapeutic technique in which the client is invited to express anger by striking cushions, shouting etc. The feelings expressed may be AUTHENTIC or RACKET FEELINGS. Feelings are often 'stacked' with the most heavily defended at the bottom so the client may move through anger into other feelings such as sadness. The most accessible feelings are often racket feelings so there is a danger that anger work will constitute stroking a racket and will therefore reinforce script and be counter-therapeutic. Some take the view that the expression of anger is itself cathartic and therefore beneficial. It is important that the client has PERMISSION to feel and to express his or her feelings appropriately, and the taking of this permission will often remove blocks to therapeutic change. It is doubtful whether the expression of anger is *in itself* helpful. Like other therapeutic interventions, anger work should only be undertaken within the framework of a treatment plan. Clients doing anger work need PROTECTION from the possible punitive response of the INTROJECT, which is the target of the anger (SCRIPT BACKLASH).

anorexia nervosa an eating disorder characterised by grossly inadequate food intake and misperception of body image (an emaciated body may be seen as obese). It occurs mainly in young women. For a transactional analysis approach to working with anorexics see Achimovich (1985), Maine (1985) and Fukazawa (1977).

anorexic suffering from ANOREXIA NERVOSA.

antiscript doing the opposite of what the script prescribes from a rebellious position. There is some disagreement about this concept, see Berne (1972); c.f. the psychoanalytic concept of REACTION FORMATION.

antisocial personality adaptation a personality structure characterised by manipulative and irresponsible behaviour. The person often presents as charming. There is usually a weak, crazy or excluded Parent. See PERSONALI-TY ADAPTATION, WARE SEQUENCE.

anxiety a state of enhanced sensitivity to threat. Unlike fear, which is focused on a specific threat or threats and subsides when these are dealt with, anxiety is characterised by a constant search for sources of threats and high and persistent AUTONOMIC AROUSAL.

appropriate behaviour behaviour that leads to problem solving and needs being met is appropriate. Inappropriate behaviour may be due to DISCOUNTING of some aspects of current reality, e.g. interpreting the world according to rules learned in the family as a child and which were never appropriate or were only appropriate to a child of a specific age *in that family*. This would involve reality being interpreted within a distorted FRAME OF REFERENCE. Inappropriate behaviour may be due merely to ignorance of aspects of current reality but usually indicates that the person is in script. Stewart and Joines (1987) define script as that part of the frame of reference that involves discounting.

archeology in transactional analysis a GAME in which therapist and client become involved in extensive investigation of the client's early experience without any clear therapeutic objectives and so avoid dealing with significant issues. In psychoanalysis this is known as the flight into history.

archeopsyche in Berne's original formulation of transactional analysis theory (Berne, 1961) a PSYCHIC ORGAN which manifests itself phenomenologically as the Child ego-state.

assertiveness verbal or non-verbal behaviour in which a person clearly expresses his or her needs and wishes and deals positively and actively with the responses of others, e.g. maintains

appropriate boundaries and insists on being heard and responded to. Assertiveness comes from Adult and is to be distinguished from aggressiveness which usually comes from Parent or Child (although aggressiveness in self-defence could come from Adult). Assertiveness training teaches techniques of assertive behaviour and is particularly directed towards people who have been trained to be over-adaptive and submissive in childhood. See OVERADAPTATION, PLEASE DRIVER, GOOD CHILD SYNDROME.

attachment the tendency to form an emotional bond with a specific person. This may be shown by a need for physical closeness and dependency on the other. The attachment theory of Bowlby (1969) stresses the importance of the attachment to the mother in the first year of life and relates adult insecurity and ANXIETY in relation to loss to failures in the mother–baby bond. Bowlby's views on the need for a bond with one person have been questioned (Rutter, 1972).

Transactional analysis stresses the importance of relationships with others through the concepts of RECOGNITION HUNGER (Berne, 1961) and STROKING (Berne, 1964) and their crucial importance for healthy child development. It also recognises the importance of the early relationship with the primary caretaker (usually the mother) through the concept of healthy SYMBIOSIS.

attribution a script message given as a statement about who the child is e.g. 'You're stupid' (direct) or 'He's not very strong' (indirect).

attunement the sense of being fully aware of the other person's sensations, needs or feelings and the communication of that awareness to the other person (Erskine, 1993). It requires an awareness of developmentally based needs and feelings, a kinesthetic and emotional sensing of the other but also requires the therapist to remain aware of the boundary between him- or herself and the client. Erskine regards this as a key factor in effective therapy. See also EMPATHY, I–THOU, INTERSUBJECTIVITY.

authentic feeling a feeling that is felt spontaneously and without internal censoring and so is congruent with experience and helpful in dealing with reality. See FOUR AUTHENTIC FEELINGS.

authority diagram see CONTRACT, THREE-CORNERED.

autonomic arousal (psychology) the autonomic nervous system deals with fight/flight responses to danger. It has two branches, the sympathetic and the parasympathetic. The sympathetic prepares the body for flight or fight, adrenaline enters the blood, digestion is inhibited so that more blood is available to the muscles, the heartbeat is speeded up and the blood vessels that supply the muscles are dilated. The parasympathic reverses this process.

Autonomic arousal refers to this preparation of the body for action.

autonomy the ability to act in response to here-and-now reality and the individual's own needs, wishes and view of reality and not to be controlled by script beliefs, the demands of an internal Parent ego-state or the views of others. Autonomous behaviour is characterised by an awareness of self, others and the world, spontaneous behaviour, open expression of AUTHENTIC FEELINGS and a willingness to enter into INTIMACY by forming respectful real:real relationships with others. Autonomy is a central concept in transactional analysis since the achievement of autonomy indicates release from SCRIPT. Treatment CONTRACTS aim to promote autonomy-related goals.

awareness the terms conscious, unconscious, preconscious and subconscious are little used in transactional analysis. Instead the distinction is made between what is in or out of awareness at a given time without postulating the existence of specific zones of the mind as in Freudian and Jungian theory.

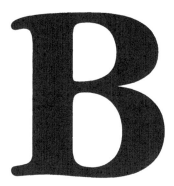

BAC British Association for Counselling. The major organisation governing counselling in the UK. It operates an ACCREDITATION scheme that is eclectic and is based on the evaluation of experience, practice and training. This scheme is therefore open to transactional analysts who have completed their training.

banal script in Steiner's (1974) classification of scripts it is a negative script (Mindless, Loveless or Joyless) that does not proceed to a dramatically bad outcome. Unlike tragic scripts, banal scripts usually go unnoticed because the banality of everyday life is so common. These are scripts of lost opportunity. Banal scripts have first or second degree PAYOFFS. Those who have banal scripts will be unhappy and unfulfilled but apparently living 'normal' lives. See also HAMARTIC SCRIPT.

basic life positions the existential positions most often taken in relation to the value of the self and others. See LIFE POSITIONS.

Be Perfect one of the five DRIVERS (Kahler and Capers, 1974). This driver is characterised by a group of behaviours including extreme precision of speech, looking upward and counting points on the fingers. The DRIVER MESSAGE directs that 'OKness' can be achieved only by getting everything right; c.f. BE STRONG, TRY HARD, PLEASE, HURRY UP.

Be Strong one of the five DRIVERS (Kahler and Capers, 1974), defensive behaviour patterns which relate to DRIVER MESSAGES. These are recipes for pleasing parents, devised in childhood and used in adult life to obtain positive feelings and to counter the negative effects of INJUNCTIONS. The drivers form an important component of the COUNTERSCRIPT. The Be Strong driver involves the person distancing himself or herself from feeling (which his or her parents had not wanted to deal with). Expression of feeling is avoided, statements about the self are generalised (e.g. 'it is cold' rather than 'I feel cold') and feelings are disowned e.g. 'you made me angry' rather than 'I felt angry when you said that'; c.f. BE PERFECT, TRY HARD, PLEASE, HURRY UP.

behavioural diagnosis of ego-states the ego-state is an internal (intrapsychic) structure but gives external signs of its presence and activity. Eric Berne (1961) described four major ways in which ego-states can be diagnosed: behavioural (what does the person do?), social (what responses do they evoke?), historical (does their behaviour correspond to some aspect of

7

their personal history?) and phenomenological (what is their experience?). For a reliable diagnosis several of these are needed, but behavioural cues are highly indicative of ego-state and can be monitored from moment-to-moment, making behavioural diagnosis a very valuable technique. Observations can be made of words, tone and speed of speech, gestures, postures, facial expressions etc. A level tone, a steady rate of speech, well-chosen words and relaxed facial muscles would indicate Adult. However, all the cues may not be congruent. Adult speech patterns with an awkward body posture or a fixed smile would probably indicate adapted Child. A diagnosis that is purely behavioural will be of the FUNCTIONAL EGO-STATE (the ego-state as it shows itself externally).

behaviourism a system of psychology, and a therapeutic technique based on it, which concentrates on behaviour rather than intrapsychic states. Classical behaviourism treated the mind as a 'black box' whose internal processes do not need to be considered as long as we understand the relationship between input and output. Modern behaviourism does take some account of mental states, and classical behaviourism has given way to a cognitive-behavioural approach. Behaviourism had significant influence on the development of transactional analysis. Its strength lay in its concern with what could be directly observed, which gave it an objectivity that psychoanalysis lacked. Classical behaviourism discounted the importance of intrapsychic processes, however. Through the concept of EGO-STATES transactional analysis links observable behaviours with intrapsychic processes and is therefore able to integrate both concepts. See CONDITIONED REFLEX, UNCONDITIONED REFLEX, REINFORCEMENT.

beliefs about self, others and the world are an important part of the FRAME OF REFERENCE (Schiff et al., 1975), the total pattern of meanings that we use to interpret our experience. The SCRIPT is the distorted part of this pattern of meanings and so includes script beliefs, beliefs that were perhaps once true for the child we were in the family we were in then, or more likely were never true but were the best sense we could make of our world then. Associated with these beliefs will be DECISIONS about how we must behave if these beliefs are true. The terms belief and decision are used extensively in transactional analysis. These are cognitive terms easily expressed in words; however, the script does not consist purely of words and thoughts, it is also held in behaviours, feelings and the body (see BODY SCRIPTING and BODY-WORK). The earlier the script element was acquired, the larger the non-verbal element it will contain. Transactional analysts are now giving more emphasis to the early acquisition of script than did Eric Berne (they are shifting from a mainly Freudian position to a more Kleinian position).

Berne, Eric, founder of transactional analysis. He was born in Montreal, Canada in 1910, the son of a doctor. After qualifying as a doctor in 1935, he moved to the US where he qualified in psychiatry. As well as practising psychiatry he began training as a psychoanalyst in 1941 with Paul Federn, who was developing the concept of ego-states. World War II soon interrupted his training and in 1943 Eric Berne, who by then had become an American citizen, joined the US Army Medical Corps. Army service exposed him to a very different culture to his psychoanalytic training. Psychoanalysis is a very slow process involving hundreds of hours of contact with each client. In the army he had to make judgements about men in little more than a minute. He discovered how much could be found out, even by such brief contact, through the use of intuition. He became interested in intuition and published a series of papers on it in professional journals. What he had discovered was that there are many cues, including body posture, tone of voice, movements, etc. that could be read to infer mental state. Psychoanalysis, with its lack of face-to-face contact and its emphasis on words, missed these. *This connection between the directly observable and the internal mental state was to form the basis of transactional analysis*. Berne's psychiatric experience had enabled him to make these connections but at this stage they were not yet fully available to him as conscious knowledge that could be passed on verbally. In 1947, just after the end of the war, Berne resumed his training in psychoanalysis, this time working with Erik Erikson. Like his previous training analyst Paul Federn, Erikson was an ego psychologist, that is he belonged to a school of psychoanalysis that stressed the importance of the way in which the client related to the outside world through the ego. DRIVE THEORY psychoanalysis, which preceded ego psychology, had laid greater emphasis on internal conflicts. Erikson was particularly interested in the development of the individual, which he saw as a lifelong process, and the societal framework in which this takes place. These were ideas he was to bring together in his major work *Childhood and Society* (1950).

Berne began to combine these ideas, intuition, ego-states, behavioural clues to internal states and Erikson's developmental and social perspectives, into a system that was soon to become transactional analysis. He also read very widely and as the system developed in his mind he incorporated ideas from many sources. He wrote a series of papers for professional journals. These set out on a highly innovative path. From the early 1950s he conducted regular evening seminars that brought together a group of professionals interested in social psychiatry (looking at psychological disturbances not purely as an individual but also as a social issue). These provided an ideal medium for developing and refining the emerging theories of the new approach that was to become transactional analysis. Meanwhile, he continued to practise as a psychiatrist and to pursue his training as a psychoanalyst. In 1956 he applied for accreditation by the American Psychoanalytic Institute but was refused. He was invited to continue with his training and reapply for membership of the Institute but decided instead to set off on a new course, to develop a new system of psychotherapy, free from what he saw as the shortcomings of psychoanalysis. By 1958 he had published articles setting out all the major transactional analysis concepts that were to be the basis of his subsequent work, but it was not until 1961 that he published his major work on the subject, *Transactional Analysis in Psychotherapy*. This remains one of the most important works in the literature of transactional analysis, giving a lucid and comprehensive account of the system, its theory, its terminology, its practice and its roots in psychoanalytic theory. In his subsequent writing Berne opened up important new areas but did not continue to set out his theory with such thoroughness. Unfortunately, it is through his later writings that he is best known, so in the absence of the theoretical base and the perspective that *Transactional Analysis in Psychotherapy* could supply, these have often been misinterpreted.

In his next book, *The Structure and Dynamics of Organizations and Groups* (1963), he moved away from transactional analysis to a review of theoretical frameworks for understanding groups including new theory which he had developed. He returned to transactional analysis in 1964 with *Games People Play*. This was aimed at a small group of professionals who were beginning to use transactional analysis. It included a brief outline of basic theory together with new thinking on a developing area of transactional analysis; the theory of GAMES (repetitive patterns of social interactions). Completely unexpectedly, the book soon became a best seller. Perhaps it was because of the combination of Berne's friendly and lucid style and his keen sense of humour. The book was an extraordinary success, being serialised in mass circulation magazines, translated into 15 languages and going though many editions. Transactional analysis was propelled from a little-known derivative of psychoanalysis to a topic of mass interest, and its founder, Eric Berne, to an international celebrity. Moreover, the book through which it was becoming known was not written for a mass audience and contained only a sketchy outline of the general theory. This had a profound effect on the development of transactional analysis and in particular on the way in which it is perceived by other professionals. Games theory was developed rapidly by Berne and other transactional analysis professionals. *Games People Play* quickly became out of date but it continued to represent what transactional analysis is about to most people. Berne's next book, *Principles of Group Treatment* (1966), was another major work embracing transactional analysis and other theoretical approaches to working with groups. It was followed by *Sex in Human Loving* in 1970, the year of his early death at the age of 60. This is a witty but rather lightweight exploration of sexual relationships in terms of transactional analysis theory. His last book, *What Do You Say After You Say Hello?*, was published posthumously in 1972 from manuscripts edited after his death. Its main theme is script theory, by then a central focus of transactional analysis. Again, he chose a colloquial title and a light, witty style to reach a mass audience, but he was also setting out his most advanced thinking. Even when being scholarly as in *Transactional Analysis in Psychotherapy, The Structure and Dynamics of Organizations and Groups* and *Principles of Group Treatment* he was lucid and witty, and even when he was aiming at a wide audience as in *Sex in Human Loving* and *What Do You Say After You Say Hello?* he could be profound.

Eric Berne has produced a radical shift in attitudes to psychotherapy. His influence goes far beyond his own school. He established an original and potent approach to psychotherapy and raised public awareness of psychological issues. He was charismatic and a great innovator and communicator. Through his writings and his personality he gave transactional analysis a meteoric start, unique in the history of psychotherapy. At his death problems remained for those who continued to use and develop transactional analysis. These included issues of identity and focus, of balancing the professional with the popular and the achievement of full professional maturity and recognition. In the quarter century since then much has been achieved.

bioenergetics a method of psychotherapy developed by Alexander Lowen based on the work of Wilhelm Reich. Reich stressed the importance of the body in holding psychological disturbance, in particular through body armouring, the tightening of blocks of muscles to create defensive structures. He developed methods of working directly on the body and an energy theory to explain his findings. Lowen has modified and extended Reich's ideas. Bioenergetics has influenced the concept of BODY SCRIPTING in transactional analysis (Cassius, 1975, 1977, Childs-Gowell and Kinnaman, 1978).

Blackstone, Peg transactional analyst. Given an Eric Berne Memorial Award in 1996 for work in the area of comparison and/or integration of transactional analysis theory or practice with other theories or practices by bridging transactional analysis and current developmental psychologies (object relations and self-psychology). See Blackstone (1993).

blamer the third position in the MINISCRIPT in which the other person is blamed from an 'I'm OK, You're not OK' position while a corresponding racket feeling (e.g. righteous indignation) is felt. In Taibi Kahler's original formulation of the miniscript this position was known as vengeful Child, however the functional ego-state may be negative controlling Parent (critical Parent) as well as negative adapted Child.

Blemish a GAME initiated from a persecuting controlling Parent position in which the other participant is undermined by constant fault finding.

Board of Certification (BOC) the body within the International Transactional Analysis Association (ITAA) responsible for the control of examinations. The corresponding body in the European Association for Transactional Analysis is known as the COC (Council of Certification).

body armouring the tensing of parts of the body such as muscle blocks as a psychological defence. A form of BODY SCRIPTING.

body language the way in which feelings and states of mind are unconsciously expressed by the posture and movement of the body. This is an important source of information for the counsellor or therapist since it is difficult to disguise and enables the therapist's insight to move ahead of what the client is prepared to disclose. To this can be added information from other non-verbal sources such as paralinguistics, e.g. speed, pitch, tone and loudness of speech. ERIC BERNE in his early work on intuition drew attention to this rich source of information that is largely left untapped by psychoanalysis. Transactional analysis traces many connections between behaviour, thinking and feeling and looks for INCONGRUITIES in which differing messages are transmitted simultaneously through different channels. Body language passes in both directions; the client is also reading the therapist. This may be used therapeutically but can also be antitherapeutic if the therapist is transmitting, out of awareness, some of their personal material. For a detailed account of the transactional analysis theory of body language, see Steere (1982).

body scripting the defensive use of the body so that elements of the script are stored within parts of the body, enabling thoughts, feelings, memories etc. to be kept out of awareness. This is discussed by Cassius (1975, 1977) and Childs-Gowell and Kinnaman (1978). For a psychoanalytic approach to this topic, see McDougall (1989). See also BIOENERGETICS.

body work working directly on the body of clients, by massage, manipulation, or inviting them to be aware of or move certain parts of their body to release BODY SCRIPTING. When this is done there may be a release of feeling or previously inaccessible memories may be contacted. Body work forms a major part of the technique of Reichian therapies such as BIOENERGETICS and Radix.

bond a strong emotional connection between two individuals which forms when they enter into ATTACHMENT.

bonding the setting-up of an emotional bond by, for example, seeking proximity or close contact, sharing activities, etc.

bound energy in Berne's energy theory (Berne, 1961) there is energy associated with each ego-state: this may be available (unbound) and then contributes to the energisation (or CATHEXIS) of that ego-state. However, it may be bound, that is potentially but not immediately available. In addition to bound and unbound energy there is also FREE ENERGY that is able to move freely between ego-states. At any given moment the ego-state that has the greatest amount of free energy is experienced as self. However the ego-state that has executive power is the one that has the greatest amount of available energy, and here the unbound energy counts too, so it is possible for the sense of self to be in an ego-state that is not actually running things (not in executive). For example, if we put most of our free energy into Adult, so we experience ourself coming from there but the remaining free energy goes to Parent and tops up the unbound energy there to the point where it takes executive power, we may watch ourselves acting in response to Parent commands, while knowing from Adult that they are inappropriate.

boundaries limits set on behaviour regarded as acceptable from others. In the counselling or therapy situation these might be on such matters as confidentiality, timekeeping, etc. Many clients have difficulty in setting boundaries. Boundaries need to be set by Adult although healthy Parent is a useful support. Angry Parent is likely to set rigid and inappropriate boundaries while the Child, particularly if the historical child was engulfed or abused, may be unable to set or defend boundaries.

bulimia nervosa an eating disorder in which there is gross overeating often followed by purging or self-induced vomiting. Bulimics have often been ANOREXIC. Unlike anorexics, bulimics often maintain normal body weight so the condition is less obvious. A transactional analysis approach to working with bulimics is discussed by Goode (1985) and Vognsen (1985).

British Association for Counselling see BAC.

bull's eye transaction a TRANSACTION (especially by a therapist) that impacts on all three ego-states (Karpman, 1971).

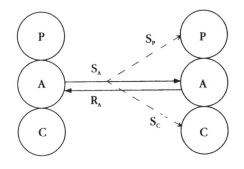

Figure 1 Bull's eye transaction (Karpman, 1971). S_A the stimulus to the Adult ego-state also stimulates the Parent and Child ego-states.

business contract that part of the therapy or counselling contract that relates to the practicalities of how the sessions should be conducted (time, place, duration, frequency of sessions, fees, etc). See CONTRACTING.

bystander (Clarkson, 1987, 1992, 1997). A fourth DRAMA TRIANGLE role is that of the bystander who watches the action and does nothing to change what is happening. By denying their responsibility and their power to act they are having a significant impact on the system. Without bystanders, oppressive systems would find it hard to operate.

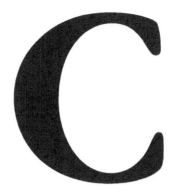

catharsis a release of emotion. The term comes from the Greek meaning 'to purge' and carries the implication that the process has a healthful, cleansing function. Such emotional releases may occur spontaneously during therapy or may be actively sought as in ANGER WORK. They often signify important points in therapy although transactional analysis warns against stroking displays of RACKET FEELINGS and thereby reinforcing SCRIPT. See also ABREACTION.

cathect to invest an intrapsychic structure e.g. an ego-state, with psychological energy.

cathexis see PSYCHIC ENERGY, SCHIFFIAN THEORY.

Cathexis School the school of transactional analysis developed by Jacqui Lee Schiff and her co-workers. This centred around the therapeutic use of REPARENTING. Other important concepts developed within the Cathexis School include DISCOUNTING, the DISCOUNT MATRIX, REDEFINING, SYMBIOSIS, the FRAME OF REFERENCE and the FOUR PASSIVE BEHAVIOURS.

chairwork see CUSHION WORK.

character disorder see ANTISOCIAL PERSONALITY ADAPTATION.

change a movement from one state to another. Clients come into counselling or psychotherapy seeking change but they are often unclear about what changes are possible or might be helpful. Transactional analysis is a contractual process in which client and therapist work together with mutual respect and agreement. In the early stages contracts may refer mainly to a joint *process* of exploration through which an understanding of the client's dilemma is developed. This then makes contracts for change possible that can be clearly specified in terms of outcomes. See CONTRACT.

Child When written with a capital this indicates the *Child ego-state*. When written with a lower case 'c' it indicates a real child.

child development transactional analysis contains many developmental concepts (the second and third order structural analysis of ego-states, the concept of the developing symbiotic relationship with the parents, etc.) but it has produced only one comprehensive theory of development, that of PAMELA LEVIN (1982, 1988). Developmental issues are profoundly relevant to the ego-state model and the script concept. The Child ego-state is not a unitary structure but an accumu-

13

lation of records of earlier patterns of thinking, feeling and behaving relating to various developmental stages. The timing of significant events relative to developmental stages is therefore very significant in terms of ego-state structure and script formation and therefore has profound implications for the individual. Berne (1961) illustrates this idea in terms of bent pennies that leave the pile permanently skewed. Transactional analysis is an integrative approach that is able to draw on other disciplines and transactional analysts draw on a wide range of theories of child development, notably those of Freud, Mahler (1975) and, most recently, Stern (1985).

Child ego-state the ego-state which holds the thinking feeling and behaviour of childhood. The transactional analysis concept of the Child ego-state has been widely influential and has been taken up by psychotherapists working within other disciplines, e.g. by the psychoanalyst Alice Miller, who usually refer to it as the *inner child*. The concept represents a major extension of psychotherapeutic theory by conceptualising the residues of earlier experience in personal form, almost as if they function as internal OBJECTS. There is not a single Child ego-state but a set of ego-states representing different developmental levels. This is represented diagrammatically in higher order analysis of ego-states by the C_2, C_1 and C_0 ego-states.

C_0 the earliest version of the Child ego-state corresponding to birth and pre-birth issues. In SECOND ORDER STRUCTURAL ANALYSIS this is shown within C_1, the early or somatic Child. According to Mellor (1986), C_0 is involved in the type 3 IMPASSE.

C_1 the early Child ego-state shown in SECOND ORDER STRUCTURAL ANALYSIS within C_2, the Child ego-state proper. This ego-state is sometimes referred to as the somatic Child as it represents a time when body issues were very important

and disturbances within this ego-state are likely to be reflected in somatic disorders. This ego-state is involved in the type 2 IMPASSE.

C_2 the Child ego-state proper representative of later childhood (about seven onwards). This ego-state is involved in the type 1 IMPASSE.

C_3 this term is sometimes used to indicate a Child ego-state within the Parent.

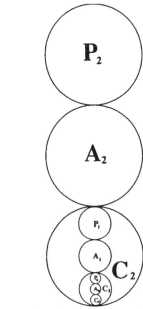

Figure 2 Third-order structural analysis of the Child ego-state. C_2 includes an earlier version C_1, which includes a still earlier version C_0.

See also EGO-STATES.

childhood memories memories of events in childhood provide important information on the way SCRIPT has been formed and provide points of connection into unassimilated early experience which are important in therapeutic techniques such as REDECISION. Memories may take many forms. Often there may be DISSOCIATION from important aspects of the original experience. Distressing events may be remembered without access to the original feelings or clients may have EXPERIENTIAL MEMORIES in the form of body sensations or moods that correspond to early experiences but are not accompanied by visual or auditory memories. The obsessive search for childhood memories without a clear therapeutic objective constitutes the game of ARCHEOLOGY.

child sexual abuse (sometimes abbreviated to CSA) the exposure of children to sexual experiences that are, or might be, damaging to their normal psychological development, usually for the gratification of an adult. This may extend from incest to exposure to pornographic material. Child sexual abuse may (and often does) have profound and complex psychological effects. It has implications for development and for relationships and may leave the Child ego-state deeply confused and set up powerful script INJUNCTIONS, in particular Don't Exist.

Clarke, Jean Illesley transactional analyst. Won an Eric Berne Memorial Award in 1996 for her contributions to applying transactional analysis to parent education. See Clarke (1978).

Classical School the work of Eric Berne and his close associates. It also includes later work developed from or closely related to this work. This includes many of the major concepts of transactional analysis e.g. EGO-STATES, SCRIPT, GAMES, STROKING and RACKETS.

client the name now preferred for someone who seeks the help of a counsellor or psychotherapist. Eric Berne used the medical term 'patient' but transactional analysts along with counsellors and many psychotherapists in other disciplines feel that this does not reflect accurately the balanced and mutually respectful therapeutic relationship that Berne did so much to promote.

client-centred therapy or counselling a name formerly used for Rogerian Therapy. See PERSON-CENTRED COUNSELLING AND THERAPY.

clinical one of the four SPECIAL FIELDS of transactional analysis. Clinical transactional analysts work psychotherapeutically with clients who present with emotional, psychological, behavioural or relationship difficulties.

Certified Transactional Analyst see CTA.

COC see COMMISSION OF CERTIFICATION.

code of ethics and practice a document prepared by a professional body such as the Institute of Transactional Analysis that specifies standards of clinical and professional practice. Reported breaches of the code can result in the implementation of a complaints procedure. A clear and demanding code and effective complaints procedure are important for the protection of the client. Like every client of a professional, the client of a psychotherapist needs to be able to rely on the therapist's expertise, skills and integrity; however, the psychotherapist's client often contacts him or her at a time of particular vulnerability. An exacting code is also of importance to the professional for maintaining public confidence. For examples of transactional analysis codes of ethics (ITA, EATA and ITAA) see Appendix 3.

codependency a situation in which a partner, consciously or, more often, out of awareness, supports a dysfunctional behaviour (e.g. alcohol dependence) in the other. By doing this they maintain the relationship in a dysfunctional way to satisfy their own dependency needs. This is characteristic of the GAMES played by alcoholics (Steiner, 1971). Both partners in a codependent relationship are attempting to maintain SYMBIOSIS.

cognitive-behavioural therapy therapeutic approaches derived from cognitive therapy and behavioural therapy. They stress the close relation between beliefs and behaviour and hold that by changing irrational beliefs it is possible

15

to reduce dysfunctional behaviour and thus achieve relief from dysfunctional feelings. The techniques of the cognitive-behavioural therapies correspond closely to what is known in transactional analysis as DECONTAMINATION.

cold pricklies in Steiner's (1974) imagery in *A Fuzzy Tale* these symbolise negative strokes.

collusion the therapist or counsellor unawarely joining with the client in supporting SCRIPT.

come on a provocation into script behaviour, often internal – 'the Parent whispering in the Child's ear'. It is often identifiable through the GALLOWS that frequently accompanies it.

Commission of Certification (COC) the body that oversees the examination and certification processes in the European Association for Transactional Analysis (EATA). The corresponding body of the International Transactional Analysis Association (ITAA) is called the Board of Certification (BOC).

communication the passage of information between individuals. Transactional analysis also sees this process occurring intrapsychically between ego-states (see INTERNAL DIALOGUE). The theory of TRANSACTIONS is essentially a theory of communication, and communication theory is implicit in much of the CLASSICAL SCHOOL of transactional analysis and also plays an important role in the work of post-classical transactional analysts such as Taibi Kahler. Eric Berne maintained the balance between the behavioural/ communications and intrapsychic approaches that is the unique stance of transactional analysis. After his death the behavioural/communications approach became dominant for a time. There was interest in the fine detail of games

resulting in large numbers of games being named and many practitioners stressed confrontations aimed at changing the communication pattern only rather than dealing also with the underlying psychological motivation. Currently the balance is swinging towards the intrapsychic leaving some of those attached to CLASSICAL SCHOOL theory concerned that insights that communication theory contributed to transactional analysis may be lost.

complaints procedure the procedure followed by a professional body when a complaint is made about an alleged breach of the CODE OF ETHICS AND PRACTICE by a counsellor or therapist. See Appendix 3.

complementary transaction see TRANSACTION, COMPLEMENTARY.

compound decision linked early decisions, e.g. 'I can exist as long as I do not get close to people'. In this example one INJUNCTION (Don't Be Close) defends against another (Don't Exist).

con the ULTERIOR TRANSACTION that invites another person into a GAME by hooking their GIMMICK (the aspect of their personality structure that makes them vulnerable to this particular psychological message). For example, the con may contain an overt or covert request for help that hooks the gimmick of someone who seeks strokes by being helpful. The game then starts in the Rescuer and Victim positions on the DRAMA TRIANGLE.

conditional stroke a STROKE with a specified or implied condition, e.g. 'I like you when you smile' or 'you look good in that red dress'.

conditioned reflex (behaviourism) now usually termed *conditioned response*. A recurring response to a specific stimulus that is the result of previous experience in which the response was reinforced (e.g. a pigeon being trained to operate a lever by being given food whenever it does so). This concept influenced the development of the transactional analysis concept of STROKING.

confidentiality an agreement that the content of therapy is private and will not be disclosed. Such an agreement is a prerequisite of the trust between counsellor or therapist and client that is essential for the creation of a THERA-PEUTIC ALLIANCE. The boundaries of confidentiality need to be clearly established in the CONTRACT that is made with the client. The client should be informed that the counsellor or therapist might need to disclose certain matters in the course of SUPERVISION and appropriate boundaries placed around that process. There may be other exceptions but these must be clearly specified and agreed. If the counselling or therapy is conducted on behalf of an agency a THREE-CORNERED CONTRACT may be needed in which each of the three relationships: client ↔ counsellor, counsellor ↔ agency and agency ↔ client is contracted for.

conflict model a model of the psyche in which different parts are seen as in conflict with each other. It is one of the most influential approaches to understanding psychological problems and is inherent in much transactional analysis thinking e.g. INTERNAL DIALOGUE, IMPASSES (see Clarkson, 1992). Freud's original PSYCHIC ORGAN model in which the ego had to mediate between the conflicting demands of the ID, the SUPEREGO and the outside world is a conflict model. See also MODELS.

confrontation literally 'bringing face to face with'. One of Berne's THERAPEUTIC OPERATIONS. It involves inviting clients to be aware of inconsistencies e.g. in their thinking and behaviour, using information previously obtained in therapy. According to Berne (1966) this throws the psyche off balance and causes a redistribution of cathexis. He warns that this may strengthen the inappropriate ego-state if the confrontation is ill timed or inappropriately worded. A heavy handed confrontation of a client, especially if there is insufficient HOLDING, is likely to push the client in the direction of not-OK adapted Child. There was a vogue for a highly confrontative style in transactional analysis in certain quarters during the 1970s. This was possibly because of two factors; the rise in the COMMUNICA-TION theory approach to transactional analysis, with a consequent neglect of intrapsychic processes, and the success the Schiffs claimed using high confrontation methods with seriously disturbed clients in therapeutic communities. The latter discounted important aspects of the Schiffs' work e.g. that it had been designed specifically for seriously disturbed clients who had little available Adult ego-state and that it was delivered in an exceptionally supportive environment.

confusion model a model of psychological disturbance in terms of confusion at some level within the psyche. The concept of confusion of the Child ego-state is central to transactional analysis theory. Confusion about the nature of reality also occurs because of CONTAMI-NATION of the Adult ego-state. See Clarkson (1992), also MODELS, REDECI-SION, STAGES OF THERAPY.

confusion racket a RACKET in which confusion is experienced substituting for a feeling that the individual does not have a PERMISSION to feel.

congruence in transactional analysis this corresponds to unanimity between ego-states so that the social message (from Adult) and the psychological message (from Child or Parent) are consistent. Lack of congruence indicates an ULTERIOR TRANSACTION. What will be observable will be inconsistencies between channels of communication (smiling while looking scared, remaining impassive while talking about something sad). It is important to check for congruence when closing ESCAPE HATCHES. If it is absent the closure is likely to be sabotaged by Child. The term congruence is also used in person-centred therapy where it designates one of Rogers' CORE CONDITIONS. The meaning here is genuineness (in transactional analysis this is called authenticity). By relating authentically, the therapist models the behaviour and invites the client to do likewise. Authenticity involves an inward contact by the counsellor or therapist with their own thoughts, feelings and body states as well as an outward contact with the client. It involves a level of risk taking, and a willingness to speak as well as understand MARTIAN.

consciousness psychoanalysis presents what is essentially a topographical view of the psyche in which the conscious, preconscious and unconscious may be seen as zones overlapping the boundaries of the PSYCHIC ORGANS. Transactional analysis traditionally has avoided using language that implies such divisions, so usually refers to psychic content (thoughts, feelings etc.) as being in or out of *awareness*. However, it is an integrative approach so transactional analysts sometimes choose to use the psychoanalytic terms.

contact (Gestalt psychotherapy) contact between the person and his or her own environment (personal and material) is seen as the basis of healthy functioning in the Gestalt approach. Psychopathology can therefore be interpreted in terms of various types of interruption to contact. This concept has been introduced into transactional analysis by Richard Erskine (Erskine and Moursund, 1988).

containment (psychoanalysis, object relations school) the therapist's taking on whatever the client offers, openly or out of awareness, and being able to deal with it safely from a mature and caring position, however disturbing it may be to them. This concept was used extensively by Bion. In Kleinian imagery it may be seen as the therapist providing a safe container for the client's PROJECTIVE IDENTIFICATION. This is closely allied to Winnicott's concept of HOLDING. In transactional analysis terms this may be seen as referring to the POTENCY of the therapist.

constant Adult a condition in which only the Adult ego-state is cathected in transactions. Similarly constant Child and constant Parent. See EXCLUSION, EGO-STATES.

contamination contents of the Child or Parent ego-states becoming confused with Adult ego-state contents (Berne, 1961). This results in current reality (the concern of the Adult) becoming confused with a past state, either a Child experience or a Parent direction or idea. This might result in an adult person feeling inadequate because that person still felt he or she had the limited intelligence and knowledge of a child, or stating an idea of a parent as if it were established fact ('you can't trust people with green eyes'). Contamination may be single (Child or Parent contamination) or double (both). The first stage of transactional analysis therapy is decontamination of the Adult to provide a resource to work alongside the therapist in deconfusing the Child.

Contamination

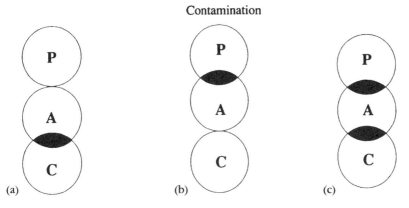

(a) Child contamination of Adult – e.g. Child belief 'spiders are scary' contaminates Adult to cause spider phobia. (b) Parent contamination of Adult – e.g. Parent belief 'all Scotsmen are mean' contaminates Adult to cause prejudice. (c) Double contamination of Adult – e.g. Parent belief 'you are a rotten kid', plus Child belief 'I am a rotten kid'.

Figure 3 Contamination (Berne, 1961).

content the material brought by the client to the psychotherapy or counselling session. What is talked about in the session. This may be clearly relevant but it also may be defensive, serving to obscure important issues and create diversion. It is important to take account also of the PROCESS, i.e. what happens in the session.

contract a negotiated agreement between the client and the therapist or counsellor. This may refer to *business* (e.g. fees, times of sessions), *process* (how the work is to be carried out) or *outcomes* (what the client seeks from the therapy). Transactional analysis is a contractual method; it stresses the importance of openness, clear communication and mutual respect. This is only possible if hidden agendas on the part of the client and the therapist are brought out and addressed. Contracting may be undertaken formally with time set aside in the session to arrive at a contract. It may also take place moment by moment in the process. This involves the therapist making frequent checks that he or she

and the client are travelling together in an agreed direction (Lee, 1997). The therapist does not have to accept the contract requested by the client; clients commonly request contracts to reinforce defences such as DRIVER BEHAVIOURS. However, the contract finally arrived at needs to be agreed by both parties without the client experiencing pressure to change in ways which the therapist believes to be 'right'. It is legitimate for the therapist to set rules that are not negotiable (e.g. no violence). These set the boundaries within which the therapy will take place and need to be clear and specific and not just assumed. The client agrees to them or does not contract to work with the therapist.

Transactional analysis stresses the importance of outcome contracts in imparting clarity to the contracting process and of specifying observable criteria by which the achievement of the contract may be assessed. The most specific criteria will be behavioural so, where possible, the OUTCOME CONTRACT specifies behaviours that will indicate the achievement of the agreed objectives. See also OUTCOME FANTASIES.

Steiner (1974) pointed out the similarities between the therapeutic process of contracting and legal concepts of contract. Contracts require mutual consent, valid consideration (both parties benefit) and competency (not only for the therapist who needs to be suitably trained and experienced, but also the client needs to have enough available Adult to participate actively in the change process). Also the contract must have a lawful object (it must not have as a goal anything that contravenes the law or the accepted ethical principles governing the practice of psychotherapy). See COVERT AGENDA.

contract, three-cornered in certain situations a third party may have an interest in the contract e.g. where counselling or psychotherapy is done within an organisation. Each of the contracts needs to be made clear, e.g. client ↔ therapist, client ↔ organisation, therapist ↔ organisation. This is known as a three-cornered contract (English, 1975). In certain situations the position is still more complex, especially if a number of individuals or bodies exercise authority but are not parties to the contracting. In this case Berne (1966) recommends the drawing-up of an authority diagram to define the space in which contracting takes place.

controlling Parent (often written Controlling Parent) the Parent ego-state functioning in a controlling mode. See FUNCTIONAL EGO-STATES.

Cops and Robbers a GAME of pursuits and evasions. Berne (1964) suggested that the person who is 'it' secretly wants to be caught, like the child who hides in Hide and Seek.

cop-out finding a crooked way out of a difficult situation. Berne (1971) sees this as a function of the Little Professor (A₁) in making the Child's adaptation to the Parent less onerous.

core conditions (person-centred counselling) those qualities expressed within the counsellor–client relationship that are necessary for effective work. Rogers (1951), within the person-centred school of counselling, identified three main core conditions which he termed, *empathy, unconditional positive regard* and *congruence.* Transactional analysis stresses the *I'm OK: You're OK position* and *authenticity* which closely correspond to Rogers' unconditional positive regard and congruence. See CONGRUENCE, THERAPEUTIC ALLIANCE, PERSON-CENTRED COUNSELLING.

corralogram a diagram that indicates the amount of time spent in each of the four LIFE POSITIONS over a period of time, usually a day (Ernst, 1971). A shape is drawn in the centre of an OK CORRAL diagram. The area covered in each quadrant indicates the proportion of time spent in that life position.

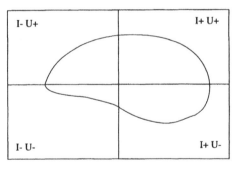

Figure 4 Corralogram (Ernst, 1971). The area of the outline falling in each quadrant of the OK Corral indicates the proportion of each day spent in that life position.

corrective emotional experience providing, within the therapy, an experience whose lack in childhood has led to a developmental failure and thus facilitating the readdressing of the developmental issue. This is rejected by some psychodynamic theorists who assert the primacy of achieving intrapsychic restructuring by analysis.

Classical transactional analysis is closer to this original Freudian position than the Cathexis and redecision schools. The emphasis in classical transactional analysis in on empowering the Adult, who can then cooperate with the therapist is deconfusing the Child (i.e. the emphasis is on restructuring rather than 'healing'). REPARENTING is based on the concept of the corrective emotional experience.

counselling currently (1997) there is a lack of agreement among transactional analysis and counselling organisations on the exact definition of counselling. A number of definitions have been proposed (e.g. ITAA, 1995). What seems to be agreed is that it is a helping activity that involves talking to others and facilitating them in processing their experience and making desired changes in their feeling, thinking and behaviour. Usually psychological theories are applied within this facilitation process. Likewise, there is no agreement that a clear distinction can be made between counselling and psychotherapy. The British Association for Counselling (1990), the major professional body for counselling in the UK, does not make a distinction between the two activities. This is a significant issue for transactional analysis as the qualification of Certified Transactional Analyst is awarded in SPECIAL FIELDS of application, which include psychotherapy and counselling. The European Association for Transactional Analysis (EATA, 1997) specifies the counselling special field as being appropriate for transactional analysts whose activities aim at the development and growth of people and their frame of reference without these activities coming under the clinical, organisational or educational field. In general those who do see a difference between counselling and psychotherapy tend to place it in the level of intrapsychic restructuring involved: 'counselling' consisting mainly of a restructuring of currently available resources while 'psychotherapy' involves deeper level interventions to make additional resources available.

counterinjunctions 'messages' acquired in later childhood that specify behaviours which the developing child believed would gain the approval (and perhaps love) of their parents. Resorting to these behaviours from an adapted Child position generates a spurious sense of OKness that helps to defend against negative elements in the personality such as INJUNCTIONS. The five DRIVER MESSAGES are important counterinjunctions that occur widely. Collectively the counterinjunctions constitute the COUNTERSCRIPT. See INJUNCTIONS, SCRIPT MATRIX, DRIVERS, MESSAGE FORMAT.

counterfeit strokes a stroke that is not what it at first appears to be – for example a negative stroke presented as a positive ('What an unusual dress! Did you get it secondhand?')

counterscript the defensive aspect of the script made up of the COUNTERINJUNCTIONS. The counterscript has a major effect on the way the script is played out since it clearly specifies behaviours (originally behaviours that the child believed would gain his or her parents' approval). The PROCESS SCRIPT type is therefore closely related to the counterscript and in particular to the principal DRIVER MESSAGES. See also SCRIPT MATRIX.

counterscript cure an apparent cure in which the client has incorporated messages from the therapist on how to be a 'good' client into his or her counterscript (Clarkson, 1992). The person is acting as if change at a deep structural level has occurred (see FLIGHT INTO HEALTH). The client has OVERADAPTED to the therapist. This should not be taken at its face value but may represent a significant stage in therapy in that the client may cease destructive behaviours and become open to the good thinking of the therapist. See also PASSIVE BEHAVIOURS.

countertransference originally the therapist's reaction to the TRANSFERENCE of the client (e.g. if the client is projecting his or her father on to the therapist he or she will elicit a response in the therapist to the psychological manoeuvres he or she has carried forward from the original situation). Awareness of countertransference yields important insights (e.g. social diagnosis of ego-states). If it is missed by the therapist then the client and therapist can be drawn into a replay of the original situation with the parent or other projected figure. This is often the cause of therapy becoming stuck and is an issue addressed in SUPERVISION. Clarkson (1992) refers to this as *reactive countertransference*. The term *countertransference* is also used to describe the therapist's transference on to the client (i.e. the projection on to the client of a significant figure from the therapist's past). Clarkson calls this *pro-active countertransference*.

Courtroom a GAME in which two parties competitively seek to secure a third person (often the therapist) as an ally against the other. Often played when couples are being counselled.

covert agenda beliefs about desired or necessary outcomes that are held by either the client or the therapist and not made explicit. If not dealt with these will give rise to ULTERIOR TRANSACTIONS in which divergent messages are given simultaneously at the social (ostensible) and psychological (real) levels. A major function of the CONTRACTING process is to make these agendas open and specific.

creative dreamer alternative term for the schizoid PERSONALITY ADAPTATION.

critical Parent (often written Critical Parent) the Parent ego-state functioning in a critical mode. This is now regarded as the negative aspect of the controlling Parent ego-state (–CP). See FUNCTIONAL EGO-STATES.

crossed transaction see TRANSACTION, CROSSED.

Crossman, Pat received the Eric Berne Memorial Scientific Award in 1976 for her work on PERMISSION and PROTECTION.

crossup see FORMULA G.

crying expressing emotion through the release of tears, often with sobbing. This may be expressive of sadness, pain or sometimes joy. Transactional analysts believe that the expression of AUTHENTIC FEELINGS is always helpful and should be supported. However, crying, along with other forms of emotional expression, may represent the expression of RACKET FEELINGS. Clients will sometimes move through the racket feelings into authentic feeling, but the STROKING of a prolonged or habitual release of racket feelings is counter-therapeutic.

crystallisation see THERAPEUTIC OPERATIONS.

CTA certified transactional analyst. A professional qualification entitling the person holding it to practise transactional analysis awarded by the relevant professional body (in Europe this is EATA, the European Association for Transactional Analysis). The CTA can be awarded in four SPECIAL FIELDS: clinical, organisational, educational or counselling. In the UK the award of CTA clinical leads to registration as a psychotherapist by the UK Council for Psychotherapy (UKCP).

cure restoration to a state of health. This has a clear meaning in medical settings but in psychology is more problematic. An intervention to reinstate defensive systems may enable the client to resume previous levels of functioning but not be in that client's long-term interests as defensive systems are limiting. A better outcome may be to help the client to function without the need for the defences. Berne (1971) stressed the importance of cure and the need to focus on the key issue and deal with it without being distracted by peripheral consequences of the pathology (he compared this to withdrawing a splinter in the toe as opposed to dealing with the limp that resulted from it). The concept of cure may be seen to run counter to the humanistic approach, which assumes an innate tendency to develop in the way that is uniquely appropriate for the individual. This humanistic perspective is also part of the philosophical position of transactional analysis. If cure is a return to (or movement towards) 'normality', who decides what is normal? The transactional analysis answer is 'the client'. In the process of CONTRACTING, client and therapist agree positive outcomes for the therapy and the ways in which these can be verified. These have to be freely agreed between them. The therapist does not seek to impose his or her view on the client but may decline to work towards an outcome that he or she believes would not be in the client's interests. See also PHYSIS.

cure, four phases of Berne (1961, 1972) proposed that there are four phases of cure.

- *social control*, in which the client takes control from Adult even though the content of the Parent and Child ego-states may remain unchanged. This may be achieved at an early stage of therapy.
- *symptomatic relief*, in which changes have begun to occur in the Child and/or Parent ego-states so there is less internal pressure to engage in scripty behaviours.
- *transference cure* A stage in which the therapist has been introjected as a good Parent. This will remain stable only if the client can maintain the introject ('keep the therapist in his or her head'). While it lasts this can give considerable relief from SCRIPT. REDECISION therapy encourages the client to stay out of TRANSFERENCE.
- *script cure* was originally called 'psychoanalytic cure' by Berne (1961). This involves a fundamental change in the Child ego-state with Adult support so that script issues can finally be resolved. See REDECISION.

curse term sometimes used for the PAYOFF of the script.

cushion work a clinical technique in which the client agrees to project an internal structure such as an INTROJECT or an EGO-STATE on to a cushion so that the internal process can be externalised. Alternatively, an empty chair may be used in which case the term 'chair work' is used. See PROJECTION, REDECISION, STUNTZ MULTIPLE CHAIR WORK.

cyclothymic subject to mood swings between elation and depression but not of such a magnitude as to lead to a diagnosis of MANIC DEPRESSIVE. The underlying ego-state structure is probably similar. For a transactional analysis therapeutic approach, see Loomis and Landsman (1980).

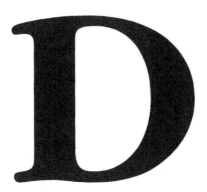

Dashiel, Sharon awarded the Eric Berne Memorial Award in Transactional Analysis in 1994 for her work on the Parent resolution process (Dashiel, 1978). (Joint award.)

decision in transactional analysis this means a choice to act or respond in a particular way made with whatever mental resources were available at the time. This term is applied to very early choices that were essentially intuitive selection of what seemed to work best as well as to later decisions that involved cognitive weighing of alternatives. See also EARLY LIFE DECISION and SCRIPT.

deconfusion the ultimate aim of transactional analysis is the deconfusion of the Child ego-state (Berne, 1961, 1972). Initially, Berne (1961) saw this stage as not always necessary and suggested that, if necessary, psychanalysis could be used to achieve it. With the development of script theory, transactional analysis developed its own approaches and deconfusion of Child came to be seen as central to achieving full script cure. See CURE, STAGES OF, THERAPEUTIC OPERATIONS.

decontamination therapeutic procedures to remove CONTAMINATION, that is to firm up boundaries between ego-states so that the Adult is free from intrusive Child or Parent material and consequently is freed from a distorted view of current reality. See THERAPEUTIC OPERATIONS.

defence mechanism (psychoanalysis) a mental process used by the EGO to control, divert or resist internal elements that may give rise to stress or anxiety ('cause neurosis'). COUNTERINJUNCTIONS are an example of a defence mechanism since they placate the internal Parent and so reduce Parent pressure on the Child. Defences are almost always associated with DISCOUNTING.

deficit a lack of something. This concept offers an alternative to trauma (damage) conflict and confusion theories of psychopathology. A problem may arise not from specific harm that the person received but from the lack of something (an experience or process), necessary for healthy development.

deficit model a model of psychological disturbance in terms of the lack of key experiences or personal resources in childhood leading to failure to complete developmental processes satisfactorily (Clarkson, 1992). See MODELS.

degree the level of pathology associated with a behaviour pattern (GAME or SCRIPT) as measured by the damaging nature of the outcome. Games played at the first degree level result in nothing more than social embarrassment; at the second degree level there are serious consequences such as loss of a job or divorce and at the third degree level they may result in psychiatric hospitalisation, imprisonment, serious physical harm or even death. See GAMES and SCRIPT.

deliberate self-harm harm to the body done in awareness (as opposed to setting up, out of awareness, to have an accident). This may extend from self-mutilation to suicide. In transactional analysis self-harm is regarded as one of the three ESCAPE HATCHES that represent ultimate and extremely damaging default strategies, which may be triggered if defences fail to hold. Closure of escape hatches (a decision from uncontaminated Adult not to use the escape hatch whatever the circumstances) must therefore precede major therapy in which important defence mechanisms are addressed. The client needs to take account of the possibility of acting out without awareness and maintain Adult awareness to prevent this.

delusion a false belief that persists despite argument, persuasion or indeed clear contrary evidence and which is not consistent with the client's educational, cultural or religious background. A delusion will involve DISCOUNTING and indicates CONTAMINATION of the Adult ego-state, usually by Child.

denial a DEFENCE MECHANISM in which a painful experience or an EGO DYSTONIC aspect of the self is denied. As with other defence mechanisms, this will be characterised by the use of DISCOUNTING.

dependency the state of needing (or believing that one needs) the support of another in order to function normally. This is a reality in childhood. A psychologically healthy adult possesses a high degree of independence but nevertheless has emotional and social needs that must be met through others. Fairbairn (1952) distinguishes between *infantile* and *mature* dependence. In this usage, mature dependence is the opposite of NARCISSISM rather than of self-reliance. For transactional analysis models of dependency see SYMBIOSIS, SECOND ORDER SYMBIOSIS, CODEPENDENCY.

depersonalisation a sense of personal unreality. This is an indicator of DISSOCIATION. See also DEREALISATION.

depression a transient mood or chronic feeling state characterised by hopelessness, despair, sadness, a sense of meaninglessness, low self-esteem and apathy. Psychiatrists distinguish between reactive depression, which has an identifiable external cause such as a loss, and endogenous depression where no such cause is identifiable and which seems to arise from internal sources. In depression people are often passive and inactive. Agitated depression is characterised by restlessness and since the sufferer has more energy the risk of self-harm is higher. Depression is always associated with a Don't Exist injunction. Other injunctions that are often present are Don't Be Important (Don't Have Needs) Don't Be You and Don't Be Well. See also MANIC DEPRESSIVE.

depressive position (Kleinian psychoanalysis) the position reached when the child (or client in therapy) leaves the PARANOID-SCHIZOID position in which there was splitting of both the EGO (self) and OBJECT representation (the way the mother is perceived) into good and bad parts, to a more realistic position in which there is awareness that both love and hate were directed to the same object. The client becomes aware of the ambivalence of the loved object (mother) and becomes concerned to make reparation for the damage he or she imagines his or her hate has done. See OBJECT CONSTANCY. This Kleinian concept influenced the transactional analysis concept of LIFE POSITION. See also OK CORRAL.

depth psychology a psychology that seeks to understand psychological problems by exploring unconscious aspects of the psyche. Psychoanalysis is such an approach. Initially transactional analysis placed major emphasis on behavioural aspects of psychological problems although its roots have always been psychoanalytic. In his early writings Berne suggested that psychoanalysis might be needed if deeper level interventions were necessary. As it has developed, transactional analysis has extended its field from relatively brief interventions (usually in a group) to include the full range of depth work. This has been accompanied recently by an incorporation of additional psychoanalytic theory, particularly later (post-Bernian) developments such as self psychology. Ian Stewart (1996a) has referred to this as a 'psychoanalytic renaissance'.

derealisation a sense that the external world is unreal. Like DEPERSONALISATION, this indicates DISSOCIATION.

destrudo (psychoanalysis) the energy associated with the death instinct or Thanatos. Berne alludes to these concepts in *A Layman's Guide to Psychiatry and Psychoanalysis* (Berne, 1957) and they may have influenced his concept of the script payoff. See also LIBIDO.

development advancing through stages to a more complex or complete state. Theories of psychological development describe, classify and seek to explain the stages of psychological organisation passed through from birth to maturity. Two widely used systems are the psychosexual stages of Freud and Erik Erikson's stages. Development may be adversely affected by DEFICITS (lack of necessary experiences) or TRAUMA (damaging experiences), which may lead to FIXATIONS (points of arrested development that may lead later to age-inappropriate thinking, feeling or behaviour). Fixations also have implications for the satisfactory completion of later developmental stages. Eric Berne compared them to bent pennies that skew the rest of the stack of coins. Transactional analysis includes many developmental concepts, e.g. the archaic nature of the Child and Parent ego-states, second order analysis of ego-states, Mellor's model of the three types of IMPASSE. The most extensive developmental model within transactional analysis is that of PAMELA LEVIN.

diagnosis the identification of a specific illness or psychological disturbance. Accurate diagnosis can lead to effective TREATMENT PLANNING; however, diagnosis can also lead to labelling in which unique aspects of the client's situation are missed and attributes that they do not have but that are associated with the label are attributed to them. Psychiatric diagnosis is based on an analogy with physical medicine: there are specific mental illnesses (e.g. schizophrenia) rather than a great variety of problems arising from the interaction of pathological factors. The overall approach in transactional analysis is one of micro-diagnosis (Feltham and Dryden, 1993), the identification of units of pathology such as a Don't Exist INJUNCTION. Since transactional analysis stresses the close connection between mental states and behaviours, these units of pathology can often be related to specific behaviours (e.g. Be Strong DRIVER behaviours). Transactional analysis also has a syndrome-based system of diagnosis, Paul Ware's concept of PERSONALITY ADAPTATIONS which is based on six characteristic patterns of diagnostic elements.

directive when the counsellor or therapist is controlling or guiding the client he or she is described as being directive. The danger lies in missing the client because the agenda has become largely that of the therapist. This also undermines the AUTONOMY of the client and contravenes the philosophical basis of transactional analysis, I'M OK, YOU'RE OK. The use of CONTRACTING, not only having a treatment contract and session contracts but contracting within the process (e.g. saying 'are you willing to . . .') is standard practice in transactional analysis therapy and helps to maintain a balanced process. It is not desirable and probably not possible for the therapist or counsellor to be truly non directive. The term was once used to describe Rogerian counselling but has now been superseded by person-centred counselling in recognition of problems in being wholly non directive. The client has a right to expect the therapist to actively pursue the therapeutic process using his or her resources fully, but also that this should be done respectfully and with MUTUALITY. For a time in the 1970s after Berne's death, a directive version of transactional analysis centring on communication theory became fashionable in certain quarters. This was often associated with high levels of CONFRONTATION. Some of the practices of Schiffian reparenting therapy were highly directive and disquiet about these contributed to the break between Jacqui Schiff and the transactional analysis movement. As a result of these historical factors transactional analysis is sometimes misperceived as a highly directive approach.

discounting (cathexis school of transactional analysis) 'an internal mechanism which involves a person minimising or ignoring some aspect of himself, others or the reality situation . . . Discounting is not operationally observable, however we can see . . . external manifestations of discounting' (Schiff et al., 1975). Discounting is an important process in maintaining the SCRIPT and dealing with threats to the FRAME OF REFERENCE. It can be manifested through PASSIVE BEHAVIOURS, REDEFINING, ULTERIOR TRANSACTIONS and behaviours from DRAMA TRIANGLE positions. Games begin with a discount (implicit in the CON and the GIMMICK) and discounting is implicit in DRIVERS. There are many readily observable indicators of discounting, although discounting is not directly observable. Discounting indicates the operation of DEFENCE MECHANISMS. The discount concept is characteristic of the use of micro-conceptualisation, identifying small behavioural indicators, which is a feature of transactional analysis. The psychoanalytic concept of defence mechanism (e.g. the defensive use of denial or projection) refers to complex patterns employing many discounts and is therefore more difficult to relate to specific behaviours.

discounting, levels of (Cathexis school of transactional analysis) discounting may occur at the level of existence, significance, change possibilities and personal abilities. See DISCOUNT MATRIX.

discount matrix (Cathexis school of transactional analysis) a table that shows the relationship between discounts in terms of generality or specificity. Working to change more specific discounts will be ineffective if more general discounts (which implicitly include the specific discount) are still in place. Discounts can be classified in four ways. There are three *areas* in which discounting may occur: self, others and the external world (consensual reality). There are three *types* of discounting: of stimuli, of problems and of options for change. In addition there are four *modes* in which each type of discounting may occur: the *existence* of stimuli etc, their *significance*, the *change possibilities* and the person's (self or other) ability to *act or react* differently. Within each area of discounting these factors interact. A discount matrix table refers to dis-counting in one area only. The most general discounts are situated towards the top left of the table, the most specific to the bottom right. The discounts are interconnected along a diagonal (each is implied by the others). In planning therapy it is necessary to identify the highest level of discounting (the highest diagonal going towards the top left-hand corner of the matrix) and work downwards diagonal by diagonal.

dissociation (also disassociation) a process in which thoughts, feelings, etc. become separated from the rest of the personality. A mild form of this may involve the recall of memories without their emotional component. Extreme forms of dissociation consti-tute dissociative disorders such as MPD

in which there is a breakdown in the usual integrated functions of con-sciousness. EXCLUSION in which an ego-state is unavailable to Adult is also a form of dissociation. The ego-state model may be considered to represent a degree of dissociation that occurs in normal functioning. Berne (1971) con-sidered the final stage of personal development to involve an integrated Adult ego-state into which valuable components of the former Parent and Child ego-states are incorporated.

Do Me Something a GAME characterised by an appeal for help from a passive position.

Don't...... messages see INJUNCTIONS.

doors to therapy Paul Ware (1983) iden-tified six PERSONALITY ADAPTATIONS each representing a syndrome of character-istic behaviours that were compatible with normal life but could be dysfunc-tional. Each adaptation has features in common with recognised psychologi-cal disorders as described in DSM-IV, and the names Ware chose for the

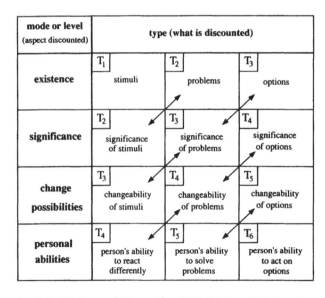

mode or level (aspect discounted)	type (what is discounted)		
existence	T_1 stimuli	T_2 problems	T_3 options
significance	T_2 significance of stimuli	T_3 significance of problems	T_4 significance of options
change possibilities	T_3 changeability of stimuli	T_4 changeability of problems	T_5 changeability of options
personal abilities	T_4 person's ability to react differently	T_5 person's ability to solve problems	T_6 person's ability to act on options

Figure 5 Discount matrix (Mellor and Sigmund., 1975). Discounting can occur in three areas – self, others and the world. A discount matrix diagram relates only to one area.

adaptations were based on the naming of these disorders (Vann Joines has since proposed other names that are not associated with psychopathology. The original names used by Paul Ware are still widely used, however). For each he identified a pattern of reaction to feeling, thinking and behaviour. One of these would be very accessible (the open door), one would be the most productive area to concentrate on in therapy (the target door), and one would be heavily involved with defensive systems and so less accessible and a potential source of trouble if addressed too early in therapy (the trap door). See WARE SEQUENCE.

drama triangle (also known as Karpman triangle) a diagram devised by Stephen Karpman (1968) on to which many patterns of interpersonal interaction (in particular GAMES) can be mapped. At the three corners are the three drama triangle positions or roles: Persecutor, Rescuer and Victim. Each is spelled with a capital letter to indicate that a drama triangle role is indicated which may differ from the everyday usage of the words. Each position is unauthentic and involves discounting. This is obvious for the Persecutor but the Rescuer is discounting the autonomy of the Victim and their power to help themselves (as also is the Victim). Rescuers are often also GRANDIOSE about their power to help others and the need for their services. Positions may be covert; it is possible to persecute from what is ostensibly a Victim position. Some people really need help and others are prepared to give it from a caring and respectful position. These authentic victims and rescuers are not on the drama triangle. As the action unfolds the participants may move round the triangle, Persecutor and Victim may change roles or the Rescuer become a Victim, etc. This movement around the triangle is characteristic of GAMES. See also BYSTANDER.

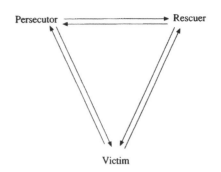

Figure 6 Drama triangle (Karpman, 1968).

dreams Spontaneous imagery occurring during sleep, which may be accompanied by other sensory modalities (hearing, touch, smell, proprioception). Freud saw them as the coded expression of unconscious processes (in particular repressed conflicts) and described them as 'the royal road to the unconscious'. In various approaches dreams are also seen as residues of daytime experience, contact with the collective unconscious or some other deep creative level of the self or even indications of the future. Berne (1972) regarded them as a mechanism for dealing with after-burn (the consequences of previous stress) and reach-back (concern over future events). Many transactional analysts work with dreams, often using techniques derived from other modalities such as Gestalt or Psychosynthesis.

dreamer see CREATIVE DREAMER.

drive theory (psychoanalysis) in the classical Freudian model of the psyche, biological instincts (e.g. sex, self-preservation) give rise to drives that are forms of psychological energy directed to seeking satisfaction of the instinct. Neurosis results from the failure of the EGO to deal with the conflicts engendered by the pressures of drives operating via the ID and the constraints of both the SUPEREGO and the outside world. In his later theories

drive theory

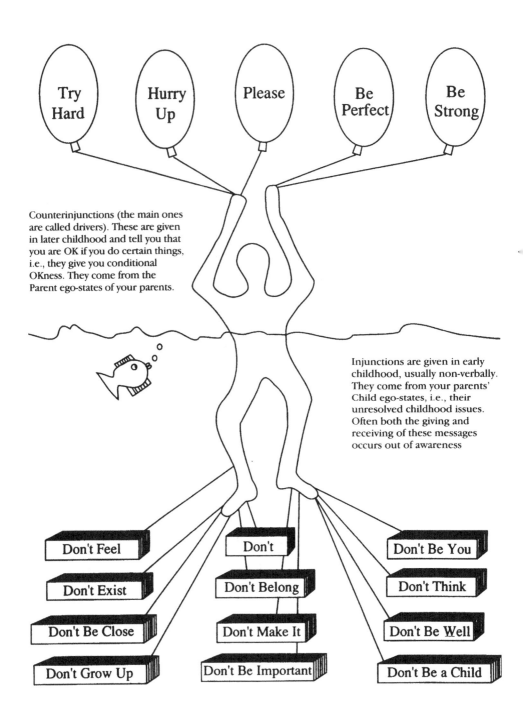

Figure 7 Drowning person (Adrienne Lee, 1988a) see page 31.

30

drive theory - continued
Freud postulated two major drives related to the life and death instincts (Eros and Thanatos). The object relations theorists shifted attention to relationships with others, in particular the mother, and internal representations of others (OBJECTS and INTERNAL OBJECTS). Ego psychology, the school of psychoanalysis in which Eric Berne trained, places greatest emphasis on the struggles of the EGO to deal with the internal and external worlds. Berne makes occasional references to drive theory concepts in his writing and it may have influenced his thinking on HUNGERS. Also the idea of SCRIPT moving towards a negative payoff is reminiscent of death instinct theory.

driver behaviour the behavioural manifestation of a DRIVER. The word driver usually implies the driver behaviour.

driver messages the implicit psychological message associated with a DRIVER. Although it is presented in MESSAGE FORMAT this does not imply that it is incorporated as a verbal message. Driver messages are COUNTERINJUNCTIONS, that is they form part of the COUNTERSCRIPT and therefore have a profound effect on the way the script is expressed in behaviours (see SCRIPT, PROCESS). In Steiner's (1971) model of the SCRIPT MATRIX they are shown as given by the Parent egostates of the parents to the Parent egostate of the client and represent beliefs about ways of achieving conditional OKness by behaving in ways that might bring the parents' approval. See also ALLOWER.

drivers brief observable behaviours, identified by Taibi Kahler (Kahler and Capers, 1974), which are indicative of underlying defensive processes. They represent responses to the COUNTERSCRIPT and carry the process of the script forwards. When a person is in driver they are dealing with internal stress arising from INJUNCTIONS (negative messages from early childhood) by engaging in behaviours which were once reinforced by parents. The process is essentially one of gaining conditional OKness by adapting to the internal Parent. See also DRIVER MESSAGE. Drivers and driver messages share the same names, which are: BE PERFECT, BE STRONG, PLEASE OTHERS, TRY HARD and HURRY UP.

Drowning person diagram a term often used to refer to Adrienne Lee's 'Scriptbound' diagram (Lee, 1988a) see page 30. This is a diagram illustrating the dynamic between COUNTERINJUNCTIONS (in particular DRIVER MESSAGES) and INJUNCTIONS in maintaining script. She was influenced by an idea of Taibi Kahler. A person is shown as attempting to stay afloat despite the weight of concrete blocks (representing INJUNCTIONS – negative messages from the past). To do this the person is clinging to balloons that represent strategies for obtaining approval learned in childhood. These give them conditional OKness ('you are OK if you do this'). The balloons symbolise COUNTERINJUNCTIONS and the messages on them are the five commonest counterinjunction messages. These five messages are also known as DRIVER MESSAGES as they are associated with behavioural patterns called DRIVERS. The diagram symbolises, in a vivid and accessible way, the most important elements of the SCRIPT MATRIX.

DSM-IV the Diagnostic and Statistical Manual of Mental Disorders. A widely used diagnostic manual published by the American Psychiatric Association. It contains an elaborate numerical and descriptive system for classifying mental disorders on the basis of their symptomatology. By concentrating on symptoms this provides a system that is, to a considerable extent, independent of theories of pathology and therefore offers a system of diagnosis that facilitates communication between professionals who have trained in differing modes of psychotherapy. For this reason it is usual to include a DSM-IV diagnosis in the case study submitted as part of the examination for Certified Transactional Analyst.

Dusay, John transactional analyst. Awarded the Eric Berne Memorial Scientific Award in 1973 for his work on EGOGRAMS (Dusay, 1972).

dynamic relating to forces. An example is Freud's psychodynamic model of psychological processes, which sees them in terms of the interplay of internal forces on the EGO (which is also exposed to pressures from the external world).

dysfunctional functioning in a way that has damaging consequences.

dystonic perceived as incongruent, inconsistent or unacceptable. See EGO DYSTONIC.

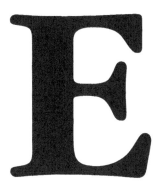

early life decision a decision taken during early childhood about the self, other people or the world that is not subsequently revised in the light of growing understanding and so becomes a basis for script formation. The word 'decision' does not imply that a high level of thinking went into the process; rather, the child needed to make choices about how to understand and deal with their world and did this with whatever mental faculties were available. Children can make decisions from the moment of birth and perhaps before. If early experiences are stressful there is less likelihood that decisions will be revised since it often feels better to have a decision that is working badly but seems to enable one to survive than to risk discarding it. Berne placed the key age of script formation at around five to seven years, following Freud's view. Many transactional analysts now agree with Melanie Klein's stress on the significance of processes of personality formation that are occurring in the first year of life.

eating disorder a psychological disorder in which there is a disturbance to normal eating patterns. Eating disorders include ANOREXIA NERVOSA, in which there is obsession with avoiding weight gain leading to gross undernutrition, and BULIMIA, in which there is binge eating followed by vomiting or purging. Eating disorders are more common in women. For transactional analysis approaches to treatment, see individual entries.

eclectic therapy a therapy that draws on a number of theoretical models. The term INTEGRATIVE THERAPY is now often preferred since the term eclectic does not exclude approaches made of random selections without an overall theory governing selection and use. Transactional analysis is an integrative approach drawing on many sources but placing them within an overall coherent theory.

ego a term used in psychoanalysis for that part of the PSYCHE or total personality which deals with the outside world and endeavours to find compromises between the demands of the ID (the source of instinctual drives such as sex), the strictures of the SUPEREGO (laying down what must and must not be done) and what is possible in the social world in which the individual finds him or herself. Classical Freudian psychoanalysis stresses instinctual drives. The psychoanalysts with whom Eric Berne trained, Erik Erikson and Paul Federn, were ego psychologists, that is they focused on ego functioning. Berne was also influenced by the British Object Relations School, especially by Ronald Fairbairn. Fairbairn (1952) divided the ego into three parts: one responded to instinctual drives, another opposed them, while a third, the central ego, dealt with the outside world. Thus the functions of Freud's three psychic organs were gathered together in the ego. This model probably influenced Berne. Transactional analysis is an ego psychology that provides a description of the functioning of the personality in terms of ego functioning.

ego dystonic a thought, feeling or behaviour is ego dystonic if it causes discomfort and is experienced as inconsistent with one's conception of oneself. See EGO SYNTONIC.

egogram a bar graph indicating the relative amounts of time spent in the five FUNCTIONAL EGO-STATES: Controlling Parent, Nurturing Parent, Adult, Natural Child (Free Child) and Adapted Child. As these are functional manifestations of ego-states this refers to behaviours, not to internal processes (which would need to be represented in terms of STRUCTURAL ANALYSIS). It may therefore not be consistent across environments (e.g. it may be different for home and work) but it is a useful way of describing personality function-

ing and identifying change strategies. It was developed by JACK DUSAY (1972) who received the Eric Berne Memorial Scientific Award for his work in 1973.

ego-state Eric Berne (1964) defined an ego-state as 'a consistent pattern of feeling and experience directly related to a corresponding consistent pattern of behaviour'. Paul Federn, who originated the idea of the ego-state, viewed it as the totality of a person's experience of himself or herself and the external world at a given moment. He suggested that past ego-states were stored in memory as totalities. Berne recognised that there were three types of ego-state: ego-states relating to past experiences of the self which he called Child ego-states; ego-states relating to past experiences of powerful significant others which he called Parent ego-states; and current ego-states relating to current experiences of here-and-now reality. He called these Adult ego-states. People would often reconnect with past ego-states and when they did they behaved as if these archaic ego-states were part of current reality. When they did so they behaved in characteristic ways that can be observed. *It is therefore possible to infer internal mental processes directly from observable behaviours.* This discovery

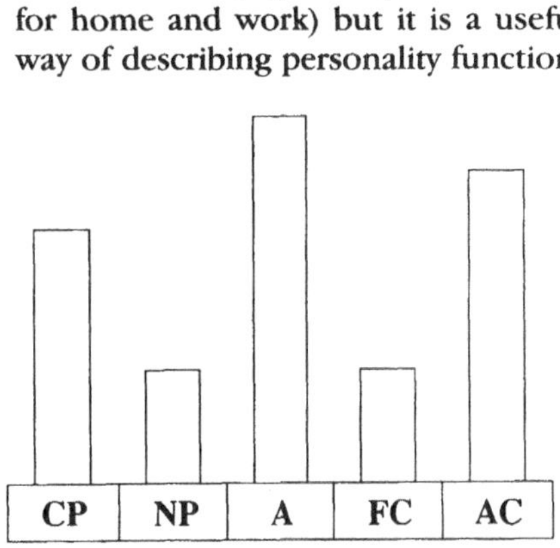

CP – controlling Parent NP – nurturing Parent
A – Adult FC – free Child (or natural Child)
AC – adapted Child

Figure 8 Egogram (Dusay, 1972).

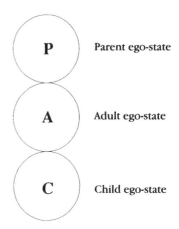

Figure 9 PAC (first-order structural analysis of ego-states) (Berne, 1961).

became the basis of transactional analysis. Berne represented each of the populations of ego-states by a circle to create a diagram of personality structure.

At any given moment CATHEXIS (psychological energy) will be directed mainly into contacting one ego-state so the person will be in a Child ego-state, a Parent ego-state or contacting 'here and now' reality through an Adult ego-state and will demonstrate this through characteristic patterns of thinking, feeling and behaviour. If a Child ego-state is contacted it will be a child of a specific age and likewise if a Parent ego-state is contacted it will be an experience with a specific parent figure at a specific time. However, once Child ego-states are selected there is a tendency to stay with them and move around between different ones in the same general area. As a 'shorthand' way of referring to this transactional analysts are inclined to say that individuals are in *their* Child ego-state or *the* Child ego-state or even 'in Child'. This is acceptable as long as one keeps in mind that it is not theoretically accurate. Usually the word 'ego-state' is omitted and the three types referred to as Parent, Adult and Child.

ego-state diagnosis Berne (1961) listed four ways of identifying ego-states:

behavioural diagnosis
social diagnosis
historical diagnosis
phenomenological diagnosis

Behavioural diagnosis is the most important as it is the most accessible. Certain behaviours are characteristic of each ego-state, e.g. diffident behaviour usually indicates Child, dominant, controlling behaviour Parent and rational, practical behaviour Adult, although each can be indicated in many other ways. Social diagnosis looks at the responses evoked in others (e.g. if these are parental the person is usually in Child).

Historical diagnosis asks 'was there a historical child or parent figure who responded in this way?' Phenomenological diagnosis asks 'what does it feel like to be in this state? Does this correspond to a past feeling state?' It is rarely possible to make a complete diagnosis on all four criteria so diagnosis is usually made mainly on behavioural grounds, using any of the other techniques that are available as checks. If diagnosis is made solely on behavioural grounds it will be of the FUNCTIONAL MODEL OF EGO-STATES.

ego-state — second-order analysis the Child and Parent ego-states are subdivided in second-order analysis. A number of parent figures will have

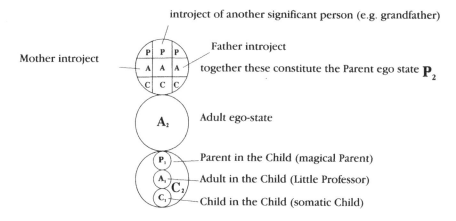

introject of another significant person (e.g. grandfather)

Mother introject

Father introject

together these constitute the Parent ego state P_2

Adult ego-state

Parent in the Child (magical Parent)
Adult in the Child (Little Professor)
Child in the Child (somatic Child)

Figure 10 Second-order structural analysis.

35

been introjected. Each of these is shown separately. Moreover, each one was a complete person with Parent, Adult and Child ego-states. These are also shown separately. The Child is subdivided to indicate early developmental stages that have contributed to its structure. It had fantasies about parental behaviour and how to have needs met by parents (corresponding to early Parent), intuitive, but not yet logical problem solving skills (early Adult) and basic child needs and wants (early Child).

ego-state – functional analysis in their behavioural manifestations the Parent and Child ego-states can show up in different ways. The Parent can seek to control others (Controlling Parent) or to look after them (Nurturing Parent). The Child can respond to the demands of its parents (Adapted Child) or to its own inner needs and wants (Natural Child – also sometimes called Free Child). This is shown by dividing the ego-state circles on the diagram. However, the division is between types of behaviour and not within the ego-states themselves. In the functional model the observer is external (the person identifying the ego-state is looking at someone else). In the structural model the observer is internal (introspectively observing his or her

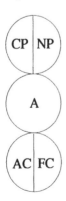

Figure 11 Functional analysis (Berne, 1961). CP – controlling Parent NP – nurturing Parent A – Adult AC – adapted Child FC – free Child (free Child is somtimes called natural Child – NC).

own mental state). See also FUNCTIONAL MODEL OF EGO-STATES.

ego syntonic a thought, feeling or behaviour is ego syntonic if it is experienced as consistent with one's conception of oneself and therefore feels comfortable.

electrode name used in some earlier TA literature for the Parent in Child (P_1) since internal messages from this usually produce a strong reaction.

empathic transactions empathic transactions involve the therapist's expression of understanding of the client's experience and the client's confirmation that she or he has been understood. This concept is inherent in the complementary transaction but had not been clearly stated in classical transactional analysis. According to Clark (1991) the continuous use of empathic transactions creates an empathic bond between the therapist and the client, making it possible for the client to feel secure enough to revive unmet needs and aborted development. The therapist is then able to reach different developmental levels of the Child to effect DECONFUSION.

empathy the power of imaginatively entering another's experience by using verbal and non-verbal information and intuition and conveying this back to the client to create a shared space in which client and therapist can work together. Empathy is stressed in person-centred counselling and is one of Rogers' CORE CONDITIONS. It is inherent in the transactional analysis concept of authenticity and AUTONOMY that implies open awareness of self and others. See also EMPATHIC TRANSACTIONS, THERAPEUTIC ALLIANCE, INTERSUBJECTIVITY.

energy psychological energy is also referred to as CATHEXIS. Berne distinguished between three types of psychological energy. Free energy is energy that can be consciously and wilfully directed to any chosen ego-state. Each ego-state also has its own potential or bound energy. This energy cannot be used until it is unbound. The ego-state with the most available energy will be in executive (i.e. be in charge of behaviour). This can be a mixture of free and unbound energy but the ego-state that is experienced as real self will have the most free energy (i.e. you will have chosen to give it the most energy).

English, Fanita transactional analyst. She received the Eric Berne Memorial Scientific Award in 1978 for her work on RACKETS, real feelings and the substitution factor (English, 1971, 1972).

episcript a negative script message that the parent passes on to the child seeking by doing so to release themselves from the influence of the message – e.g. a Don't Exist injunction is passed on to the child by a parent. Such transmission can cascade down several generations. Also called a 'hot potato' (English, 1969). This can be considered a form of PROJECTIVE IDENTIFICATION.

Eric Berne Memorial Awards the Eric Berne Memorial Scientific Award was established in 1971 in memory of Eric Berne who had died the previous year. It was given annually to the originator of a new scientific concept in transactional analysis. In 1990 the title and scope of the award was changed. It is now known as the Eric Berne Memorial Award in Transactional Analysis and is awarded annually for published contributions to transactional analysis theory or practice, or the integration or comparison of transactional analysis theory or practice with other therapeutic modalities.

Ernst, Franklin received the Eric Berne Memorial Scientific Award in 1981 for his work on the OK CORRAL (Ernst, 1971)

Erskine, Richard received the Eric Berne Memorial Scientific Award in 1982 jointly with MARILYN ZALCMAN for their work on the RACKET SYSTEM and racket analysis. Richard Erskine has also worked extensively on integrating transactional analysis with other therapeutic modalities, in particular self psychology and object relations psychoanalysis and also Gestalt therapy. See Erskine and Moursund (1988) and Erskine and Trautmann (1993).

escape hatch the Child's three options 'if things get bad enough I can always/kill myself/blame someone else and kill them/go crazy' are called the three escape hatches (Holloway, 1973; Cowles-Boyd, 1980). While these remain open there is the risk that the script will lead to a tragic outcome at some crisis point. While energy remains invested in them they are also a major obstacle to script change since they represent a mechanism for evading responsibility for making life changes (at the back of the mind there is the thought 'if things get bad enough I could always . . .'). Psychotherapy involves the dismantling of defensive structures such as COUNTERINJUNCTIONS or INJUNCTIONS that form part of a COMPOUND DECISION. This may expose damaging early decisions such as 'I have no right to exist' and increase the risk of tragic outcomes. Transactional analysts therefore consider it essential to close escape hatches before doing major change work such as REDECISION. Closure involves the client deciding from Adult to give up the escape hatch options with the therapist acting as a witness. *Promising* to close escape hatches is an adapted closure that is unlikely to hold under stress. Escape-hatch closure is an important way in which clients are given PROTECTION. Sometimes clients are unwilling to close escape hatches but are able to decide to do so for a limited period. This may be sufficient for essential work to be done safely. Time limited closure of escape hatches is sometimes referred to as *soft closure.*

ethics the philosophy of moral behaviour. The system of principles and rules that specify what constitutes good behaviour and what does not. A rule is specific and therefore easier to apply but may prove narrow and rigid. Principles are more general and closer to underlying philosophy but are more difficult to apply in specific cases. Professional bodies such as the Institute of Transactional Analysis formulate codes of ethics and professional practice to guide their practitioners which contain a balanced mixture of rules and principles. See the examples of codes of major transactional analysis organisations in Appendix 3.

euhemerus a figure from the past who has acquired a particular positive significance for a group (Berne, 1963). Berne has this role in transactional analysis.

exclusion a situation in which one ego-state (Parent, Adult or Child) constantly dominates, resulting in a stereotyped, predictable attitude, which is maintained as long as possible in any threatening situation (Berne, 1961). The dominant ego-state is referred to as *excluding* Parent, etc. This may be seen in terms of DISSOCIATION or of concentration of CATHEXIS in a single ego-state and has a defensive function.

executive the ego-state, which is able to determine a person's actions is said to be in the executive. In Berne's (1961) ENERGY theory the ego-state that has the largest total of unbound and free energy is in the executive. However, the sense of self rests with the ego-state which has the largest amount of free energy; therefore people sometimes behave in ways that they perceive as EGO DYSTONIC.

experiential memory a memory that manifests itself through body states, emotional experiences or moods without visual or auditory components necessarily being involved. See UNTHOUGHT KNOWN.

explanation see THERAPEUTIC OPERATIONS.

exteropsyche in Berne's (1961) theory of ego-states the PSYCHIC ORGAN that manifests itself phenomenologically as the Parent ego-state. See also ARCHEO-PSYCHE, NEOPSYCHE.

extrovert (Jungian analytic psychology) A personality type characterised by a tendency to direct energies outwards to the physical and social environments. People with this type of personality are often described as lively and outgoing. See also INTROVERT. In Paul Ware's personality theory the extrovert is likely to be placed in the HISTRIONIC PERSONALITY ADAPTATION.

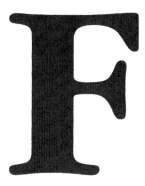

facilitator someone who enables a process to occur more readily. Often used in preference to 'therapist' for the person taking the active role in a group or workshop where the objective is personal development rather than intrapsychic change.

Fairbairn, Ronald Scottish psychoanalyst of the Object Relations school. His work was known to Berne and probably influenced him.

false self (psychoanalysis — object relations) term used by Winnicott (1971) to describe a situation where a child does not grow to acknowledge and respond to his or her own feelings. Because the mother has failed to respond to them the child has had to shift from being centred on his or her own being and needs to be concerned for the mother from whom help is needed. This creates a flaw in the structure of the self and a false self that is centred on the needs and expectations of others. This closely resembles the transactional analysis concept of the ADAPTED CHILD; however, this is a functional concept (i.e. it relates to observable behaviours and not necessarily to intrapsychic structure). See also SECOND-ORDER SYMBIOSIS, PLEASE DRIVER.

fantasy internal imagery and story telling. Fantasies may be used to main-

tain the script (see SCRIPT SYSTEM) e.g. by being used to elicit RACKET FEELINGS without involvement with here-and-now reality. All plans for the future are fantasies and our ability to fantasise is enormously valuable. Positive fantasies, e.g. of feeling and behaving differently, are useful aids for change. See also AFFIRMATIONS, PHANTASY.

father the male parent or anyone who takes the paternal role (who may not be biologically related to the child, or even not male). Although, like the mother, this is a nurturing role towards the child, the father has an important role in supporting the mother as she takes the major role in caring for the child. In the past, in Western society, the father was often seen as the parent with the strongest links into society outside the family. The object relations theorist Donald Winnicott used the term NURSING TRIAD for the system of father, mother and child. Failure to create this supportive system can result in the mother turning to the child for emotional support, thus setting up SECOND-ORDER SYMBIOSIS.

fear one of the FOUR AUTHENTIC FEELINGS recognised by transactional analysis (an authentic feeling is one that motivates the individual to deal with current life problems). Fear is a feeling that motivates the individual to avoid danger. Unlike anxiety, fear is valuable. It differs in being focused on to specific dangers, thus motivating present action to avoid future harm. Anxiety is an unfocused state of arousal that seeks unspecified threats. Appropriate arousal in dangerous environments is useful but anxiety is often disabling and may not relate to current dangers. By focusing on specific dangers, fear leads to problem solving but anxiety does not.

Federn, Paul American psychoanalyst with whom Berne trained from 1941 to 1943. Both he and Erik Erikson, the training analyst with whom Berne worked subsequently, adopted an 'ego psychology' approach that stressed the function of the ego in dealing with the outside world over the internal struggle with instinctual drives which was central to classical DRIVE THEORY psychoanalysis. Both the ego psychology approach and Federn's concept of the ego-state were important influences on Berne.

feeling also called emotion or affect. Transactional analysis distinguishes between AUTHENTIC FEELINGS, which lead to engagement with current life issues, and RACKET FEELINGS, which involve replaying past issues and adaptations. It recognises FOUR AUTHENTIC FEELINGS.

feeling loop a system developed by Moiso (1984) for analysing the processing of feeling that integrates many ideas including rackets, games, instinctual processes, neurological systems and the tendency to seek closed GESTALTEN.

fees agreement on fees forms part of the BUSINESS CONTRACT between the client and the therapist. In Steiner's (1974) terms (based on the legal concepts of contracting) fees constitute a *valid consideration* and serve to symbolise an equal exchange between client and

therapist in which each gives something of value to the other. See CONTRACT.

Ferenczi, Sandor psychoanalyst. Although close to Freud he advocated a much more involved style of working which took account of the fact that the therapy situation is a two-person system in which both TRANSFERENCE and COUNTERTRANSFERENCE are significant. He believed that the client reacted to the real personality of the analyst (Freudian psychoanalysis advocated that the analyst be distant and serve as a 'blank screen' to receive projections). He saw therapy as giving the client the opportunity to relive his or her experiences in a more permissive and supportive atmosphere. As Melanie Klein's analyst he influenced the OBJECT RELATIONS SCHOOL and he may have been an influence on Berne as transactional analysis is one of the few two-person approaches to psychotherapy and is practised in an involved and supportive style.

first-order diagram a diagram of the ego that shows it divided into Parent, Adult and Child ego-states but is not further subdivided. It is sometimes called the PAC diagram.

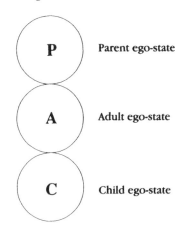

Parent ego-state

Adult ego-state

Child ego-state

Figure 12 PAC (Berne, 1961).

first rule of communication one of Berne's (1964) three RULES OF COMMUNICATION. It states that 'so long as the transactions remain complementary communication can continue indefinitely'. *'Complementary* transactions' means that the ego-state that replies is the one that is addressed and the reply is addressed to the ego-state that initiated i.e. both people are agreed as to who shall be in which ego-state. An example would be a stimulus Parent to Child responded to Child to Parent. When illustrated the vectors run parallel.

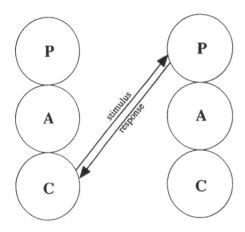

Figure 13 Complementary transaction (Berne, 1961).

five chair work see STUNTZ MULTIPLE CHAIR WORK.

fixation (psychoanalysis) a fixation represents a failure to progress through a stage of development (ambivalent attachment to an OBJECT appropriate to an earlier stage of development). Fixation results in reversion to earlier behaviours, especially when under stress, as if seeking to resolve an earlier conflict through re-enactment. Consequent internal conflict may cause the person to suffer from lack of energy. Berne (1961) uses the analogy of a bent penny that skews the pile of pennies placed on top of it. Likewise a

fixation, being an unresolved developmental issue, does not provide a firm base for subsequent development and may be a factor in later developmental failure. Fixation may also be seen in terms of a deficit in something needed to complete the developmental process. Levin (1982, 1988) is particularly associated with this approach in transactional analysis.

flight into health (psychoanalysis) the client seeks to terminate therapy on the grounds that he or she is cured although not appearing to others to have dealt with the fundamental issues. In transactional analysis this represents COUNTERSCRIPT CURE in which the client has adapted to the therapist (learned how to be a good client).

flight into history (psychoanalysis) an excessive preoccupation with past events to the exclusion of current issues in therapy to avoid internal conflict. If the therapist colludes then client and therapist play the game of ARCHEOLOGY.

flight into illness (psychoanalysis) the use of psychological symptoms to escape from internal conflict. The ploy 'How can anyone with a problem like mine be expected to . . .' may be used to avoid situations that might expose internal conflict. The game of WOODEN LEG ('how can anyone with a wooden leg be expected to dance the jig?') is based on this manoeuvre.

forming Tuckman's (1965) first stage in small group formation in which provisional groupings of members are established and members form (in Berne's 1963 terminology) a provisional GROUP IMAGO. See GROUPS, STAGES OF DEVELOPMENT.

formula G a formula used by Berne (1972) to describe the sequence of moves in a GAME. Berne repeatedly

41

refined his definition of a game. As the concept became more clearly specified, behaviour patterns previously classified as games were excluded. Many of the games described in *Games People Play* are in this category. Formula G was Berne's final definition of a game and appears in his last book, *What Do You Say After You Say Hello?* (Berne, 1972). Formula G states that in a game the following sequence of events will be observable:

CON + GIMMICK = RESPONSE → SWITCH → CROSSUP → PAYOFF

or expressed as a formula

$$C + G = R \rightarrow S \rightarrow X \rightarrow P$$

The con is the invitation given by the person who makes the first move. The gimmick is the aspect of the other party that makes him or her vulnerable to the con. The response is the social process that ensues, most of which is ostensibly Adult although involving ULTERIOR TRANSACTIONS. This may continue for seconds, hours, days or years but if the sequence is a true game at some stage there will be a series of rapid changes. At the switch each player (there may be more than two) changes ego-state and drama triangle position, e.g. the Rescuer may start to persecute, there will be a moment of confusion (the crossup) and each participant will experience RACKET FEELINGS (the payoff). The last three stages may be, in effect, simultaneous.

formula S a formula suggested by Berne to outline the main features of SCRIPT. It has been largely superseded by later developments in script theory.

four myths Taibi Kahler (1978) suggested that four myths underlie DRIVERS and RACKETS. These comprise two pairs of a negative Parent message and an adapted Child response:

(—NP) I can make you feel good by doing your thinking for you.
(AC) You can make me feel good by doing my thinking for me.
(—CP) I can make you feel bad by what I say to you.
(—AC) You can make me feel bad by what you say to me.

When we get into drivers and rackets while communicating we are replaying these internally.

four passive behaviours Schiff et al. (1971) describe four passive behaviours. Each involves avoiding problem solving in the here-and-now (although energy may be discharged inappropriately). They DISCOUNT the individual's ability to act positively to have their needs met. The four passive behaviours are:

doing nothing

overadaptation (this involves complying with a Child belief about what the other person wants without checking)

agitation (purposeless, repetitive behaviour to discharge tension)

incapacitation or violence (energy is turned inward against the self or outwards against others instead of being put into problem solving).

When working with passive clients, inviting them into overadaptation may offer a route forward in that the client becomes actively responsive to the therapist who can then invite them into authentic behaviour.

four authentic feelings sadness, anger, happiness and fear ('sad, mad, glad, scared') are feelings which, if expressed in a healthy and supportive environment, lead to solving problems and getting needs met. Each has an appropriate context and an appropriate time frame. Each of the authentic feelings can also be expressed unauthentically as RACKET FEELINGS.

Sadness relates to loss of someone or something one has been attached to; its time frame is therefore the past. Expression of sadness is an important part of mourning, a letting-go of the past so that new attachments can be made, and invites others to offer support in that process.

Anger relates to a sense of not being well treated in the present and provides energy to engage actively with others to get this changed. If anger is not discharged in the present process (is taken out of its appropriate time frame), particularly if it is saved (see STAMPS) it may reach excessive levels and be damaging rather than helpful. This sometimes leads to anger being classified as a 'bad' feeling.

Happiness indicates that all is going well with your life and you do not need to make changes. Like anger its time frame is the present.

Fear's time frame is the future (and sometimes also the present). It is a response to some dangerous situation that is about to happen or is anticipated in the future. If some action can be taken in the present to make the future safer then this is a helpful feeling. Expression of fear invites others to help you do this. If fear is focused solely on the future (e.g. on a hypothesised future event that cannot be guarded against in the present) it is likely to be a RACKET.

frame of reference this term was used by Schiff et al. (1975) to describe an individual's unique way of seeing the world. This integrates the totality of our experiences, beliefs and expectations and determines what we see and how we see it, and also what we

fail to see or DISCOUNT. It influences the meanings we give to our experiences and therefore what we feel and do. This definition resembles that of SCRIPT. According to Stewart and Joines (1987) script consists of all the definitions in the frame of reference that entail discounts, therefore the frame of reference includes the script.

free Child (often written Free Child) in the FUNCTIONAL MODEL OF EGO-STATES this refers to the aspect of the Child ego-state which has not submitted to the controlling influence of the parents and other authority figures. Sometimes referred to as natural Child.

free energy in the energy theory of Berne (1961), that part of the charge of psychological energy or cathexis which is able to move freely between ego-states. Energy may also be *bound* (held unavailable in an ego-state) or *unbound* (available but only within its specific ego-state). See ENERGY.

frequency of therapy sessions this is one of the matters dealt with in the THERAPY CONTRACT. Many variations are possible. Weekly one-hour individual sessions are common in transactional analysis. Group therapy sessions may last up to three hours and are also usually weekly. One-off extended group sessions that may last up to several days are known as MARATHONS.

Freud, Sigmund Austrian neurologist. The founder of psychoanalysis. Freud's work has been the foundation of modern psychotherapy and had a profound influence on most of the major schools of therapy. Eric Berne trained as a psychoanalyst and many of the concepts of transactional analysis have their roots in Freud's thinking.

frogs into princes (and princesses) according to Berne (1972), all children are born princes or princesses but negative parental influences often turn them into frogs. It is the business of the psychotherapist to help break the spell.

functional (model of) ego-states a model of ego-states that stresses the ways in which they manifest in interpersonal interactions. The emphasis is on the external social frame rather than the internal intrapsychic frame that is dealt with by using the STRUCTURAL MODEL. The Parent and Child ego-states are able to function in distinctive ways. The Parent ego-state may be *controlling*, demanding certain behaviours, setting limits, stating rules, being critical, etc. or it may be *nurturant*, offering support, care and protection. The Child ego-state may

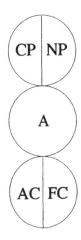

Figure 14 Functional analysis (Berne, 1961). CP – controlling Parent NP – nurturant Parent A – Adult AC – adapted Child FC – free Child (free Child is sometimes called natural Child – NC).

be *free*, natural and spontaneous, expressing feelings and seeking to get its own needs met, or it may be *adapted*, responding to the demands and needs (real and imagined) of parents or other significant people (see also FALSE SELF). Each of these states tends to be fairly stable and is represented on the functional ego-state diagram as subdivisions of the Parent and Child ego-states. Controlling Parent is abbreviated CP, nurturing Parent NP, free Child FC (also sometimes written natural Child NC) and adapted Child AC.

Other terms used to describe functional ego-states are:

• Critical Parent: this is now referred to as negative controlling Parent.
• Rebellious Child: this was often treated as a separate functional ego-state but is now regarded as a subdivision of the adapted Child. Behaviour is still regulated by perceived Parent messages but the response is negative instead of positive. The positive response can be specified as compliant Child.

There is some confusion in the transactional analysis literature as to whether functional ego-states are true ego-states. Some authors appear to treat them as if they are, for example Karpman (1971) and Goulding and Goulding (1979) in their formulation of the type three impasse. This confusion probably derives from the integrative nature of transactional analysis that has integrated both behavioural (external observer) and intrapsychic (internal observer) viewpoints. The concept of functional ego-states is an extremely useful tool for describing patterns of behaviour that are clearly linked to ego-states, but the criteria for identifying a functional ego-state are far less rigorous than those specified by Berne (1961) for the firm identification of an intrapsychic ego-state, which requires the use of historical, social and phenomenological diagnosis in addition to behavioural. In formulating theory the viewpoint is often primarily intrapsychic so the functional ego-state concept needs to be used with caution.

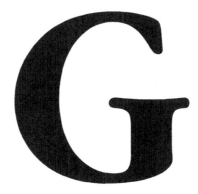

gallows see GALLOWS LAUGH.

gallows laugh laughing when making a statement about something unpleasant. The laugh is incongruent with the content of the words and invites the listener to reinforce a script belief by joining in the laugh. For example a person who tells the story of a mistake he or she made and ends by saying with a laugh 'that's just like me, I never get things right'. He or she is inviting the listeners to join in the amusement and confirm his or her script belief: 'I can't think'. Also *gallows smile* and *gallows transaction*. These terms are often abbreviated to *gallows*. Gallows is indicative of DISCOUNTING. The origin of the term is the highwayman who dies laughing at his own misfortune and is in effect saying internally: 'Well, mother, you predicted I would end up on the gallows and here I am!' See also LAUGHTER.

game formula a formula that sets out the characteristic sequence of events in a GAME. See FORMULA G.

game plan a systematic procedure for elucidating games developed by John James (1973). In outline it consists in finding answers to the following questions:

- What keeps happening over and over again?

- How does it start?
- What happens next?
- And then what happens?
- How does it end?
- And how do you feel after it ends?

Exploration of each of these issues leads to identification of DRAMA TRIANGLE switches and FORMULA G stages of the game.

games Repetitive patterns of social behaviour which are characterised by ULTERIOR TRANSACTIONS (transactions operating at two levels, an acknowledged *social* level and an unacknowledged *psychological* level) and ending with the parties feeling 'bad' (i.e. experiencing RACKET FEELINGS) (Berne, 1964). In psychodynamic terms they involve TRANSFERENCE and the ACTING OUT of unresolved archaic issues. The concept of games evolved over time and this is reflected in a variety of definitions in the literature although all fall within the criteria given above. In Berne's writings the definition increased in detail and precision so that his final definition (a sequence that includes all the stages of FORMULA G) excludes many of the patterns labelled as games in *Games People Play*. Some contemporary transactional analysts prefer a more general definition of games than this version; however, Berne's early definition did not include the *switch* and therefore failed to distinguish game playing from RACKETEERING.

Although games involve the manipulation of others through unauthentic behaviour and feeling, they are not operated from a position of awareness. Conscious manipulation of others is not a game in the sense that the word is used in transactional analysis. Although when viewed from the outside games appear to be highly negative, they do bring social and psychological advantages (see ADVANTAGES OF GAMES). Game playing is based on responding to early beliefs about available ways of getting needs met and about self, others and the world – i.e. they form part of the FRAME OF REFERENCE. Games also help to meet STROKING and TIME STRUCTURING needs (although in a very unsatisfactory way). Unless these aspects are taken into consideration direct confrontation of a game is likely to be ineffective.

games, advantages of (reasons for playing) Berne (1964) listed six advantages of games:

1. The internal psychological advantage: games help to maintain script beliefs. Although script beliefs are in reality archaic and unhelpful, to the Child they represent ways of understanding and dealing with the world. If they remain unchallenged the world remains predictable.
2. External psychological advantage: they enable situations that would be difficult to deal with (that would challenge the FRAME OF REFERENCE) to be avoided.
3. Internal social advantage: Berne (1964) wrote '[games] offer a framework for pseudo-intimate socialising indoors or in privacy', that is they result in people becoming closely involved with each other but in an unauthentic way involving ulterior transactions.
4. External social advantage: gaming gives us something to talk about.
5. Biological advantage: gaming yields strokes, even though most of them are negative. Many people find in childhood that negative strokes are the easiest to get and learn to seek them to avoid stroke deprivation.
6. Existential advantage: games generate experiences that can be used to reinforce the LIFE POSITION. As with advantages 1 and 2, this helps to maintain a familiar world view and reassures the Child. This is done particularly through the PAYOFF, the release of racket feelings at the end of the game.

In terms of Schiffian (Cathexis school) theory, games represent an attempt to maintain SYMBIOSIS (to hang on to unresolved symbiotic relationships by re-enacting them). In order to do this they have to DISCOUNT many aspects of current reality. Both the con and the gimmick that initiate the game involve discounts, and further discounting occurs as the game proceeds. In the process of the game each participant takes up a symbiotic role. This can be related to the DRAMA TRIANGLE. Persecutors and Rescuers take up a Parent position and Victims a Child position. At the crossup the positions are exchanged.

In terms of classical psychoanalytic theory, games represent ACTING OUT of unresolved unconscious conflicts and involve a transferential replay of earlier situations. See REPETITION COMPULSION.

In terms of Kleinian psychoanalytic theory games may be understood in terms of PROJECTIVE IDENTIFICATION, the con being the mechanism of projection and the gimmick that aspect of the person who is drawn into the game that makes them vulnerable to the projection. The switch occurs when the projection is disowned. This would suggest that the con may at times be very subtle and not a clearly identifiable behaviour pattern. The withdrawal of the projective identification will leave the initiator of the game with a major issue undefended, thus the move into RACKETS and often the immediate initiation of another game. At this stage there may be the maximum level of escalation in an attempt to force the other back into interaction. The limits set by the participants to escalation determine the DEGREE (level of manifest pathology) of the game. In this view, successful confrontation of games will depend on there being sufficient CONTAINMENT for the issue that was being defended by the projective identification. RACKETEERING can similarly be understood as ongoing projective identification.

games, bilateral nature of Hine (1990) pointed out that game analysis in terms of FORMULA G is focused on the initiator of the game. Although Berne (1964) defined games as 'an ongoing series of complementary transactions' this one-sided view of games has sometimes obscured the fact that both participants are playing a game and *these are different and complementary games*. For example, if one is gaming from a Persecutor position, at the same time the other must be gaming from a Victim position. Hine formulated an alternative version of formula G to represent this. She also proposed that the discharge of negative energy that occurs in the payoff is likely to initiate fresh gaming so that the gaming process is both bilateral and ongoing.

games, degrees of games are classified as first, second or third degree according to level of social damage involved in the payoff. A first degree game will cause social embarrassment, a second degree game will have major consequences such as the loss of one's job whereas a third degree game will result in such consequences as major violence, hospitalisation or imprisonment.

games, naming of in the early development of games theory there was an emphasis on behavioural analysis so that games that were expressed in significantly different behavioural patterns were given different names. This resulted in the naming of a large number of games. Emphasis has shifted to underlying processes and the identification of a relatively small number of game patterns that are given the name of a typical member (e.g. NIGYYSOB is a typical Persecutor game). The names chosen have been colloquial and humorous, often vividly and simply portraying the process of the game. This has made them easy to remember and use. The names can also sound disparaging. The word 'game' itself can also be heard in this way with its associations with conscious manipulation (although it is not used in this sense in transactional analysis).

Games People Play Eric Berne's second book on transactional analysis first published in 1964. It followed his major work *Transactional Analysis in Psychotherapy* and contains a brief account of transactional analysis followed by an exposition of the then newly developing field of game theory. It was designed to enlighten (and amuse) a small group of professionals, but thanks to Berne's lucid, accessible and engaging style it had an extraordinary success, achieving best-seller status in many countries. This brought transactional analysis to the attention of a very wide public. Regrettably, it is often the only book on transactional analysis that many people know, but as it contains only a brief exposition of general theory and games theory has developed extensively since it was written, its success has brought both fame and misunderstanding to transactional analysis.

games, relation to script games involve the reinforcement of many aspects of script e.g. script beliefs, life position, drivers, rackets, patterns of discounting, frame of reference etc. They form a large part of the interactions through which the script is maintained and moved forwards.

genogram a diagram representing family relationships often extending over several generations. It is valuable in transactional analysis to trace the handing down of script elements such as beliefs and INJUNCTIONS (see also HOT POTATO). It serves also to access feelings over family relationships and is of particular value in couples and family therapy.

Gestalt (plural Gestalten), complete a complete pattern of thoughts, feelings and responses, for example where a need has been recognised and expressed and has received an appropriate response. This Gestalt therapy term is widely used in transactional analysis.

Gestalt therapy Gestalt is an holistic/humanistic psychotherapy founded by Frederick (Fritz) and Laura Perls on the 1940s. They named their approach after the German word meaning 'whole' or 'complete pattern'. Kurt Lewin's field theory was an important influence. Taking account of the person's perceptual field (internal and external) a certain stimulus or group of stimuli will stand out and become the focus of attention (in Gestalt terminology this is the *figure*). This may be outside or inside oneself. The rest of the stimuli will recede into the background and become what is known in Gestalt as the *ground*. Once the demand represented by the figure stimuli is dealt with then energy is free to deal with the next demand. For example on returning from a walk in the country you may be cold, hungry and have wet socks. Cold may first become figure and be dealt with by sitting near the fire. Hunger then moves out of ground and becomes figure and you get something to eat. This demand having been met you then

become aware of the wet socks. It is this ability to adjust dynamically and spontaneously in the here-and-now that is equated with health by Gestalt therapists. When demands are not dealt with, energy can remain tied up with 'unfinished business' from the past. Energy is then unavailable for here-and-now demands. Energy tied up in one part of the self can also be in opposition to other parts of the self. The important Gestalt technique of TWO CHAIR WORK facilitates dialogue between these parts. This technique has been adopted by transactional analysis and is central to the REDECISION SCHOOL (Goulding and Goulding 1979). One of the major methodologies in Gestalt is focusing on bodily, emotional, cognitive and other processes in order to increase awareness. Another involves experimenting with new and different courses of action. New awarenesses lead to new actions, and new actions lead to new awarenesses. With full awareness we can choose our course of action. This is where Gestalt's roots in the phenomenological approach is evident. The quality of contact between therapist and client is also important. Martin Buber (1970) wrote of the 'I-Thou', a meeting in which two or more self-responsible human beings retain a respectful attitude and relate authentically with each-other without pretence. It is this attitude which Gestalt therapists aim to maintain with clients, believing that contact of this kind is healing in itself. Gestalt therapy has had important influences on transactional analysis. In addition to its major influence on the REDECISION SCHOOL it has also had an extensive influence on Richard Erskine's INTEGRATIVE approach and has influenced the way in which transactional analysis is practised. (See also TRANSACTIONAL ANALYSIS, SCHOOLS OF and PHENOMENOLOGY).

gimmick the aspect of a person who gets drawn into a GAME that makes them vulnerable to the CON or invitation from the other party. See FORMULA G.

good child syndrome a term used by Weiss and Weiss (1984) to describe a situation in which a person seeks to have his or her needs met by being 'good' (seeking to please others by guessing what they want and giving it to them without their having indicated that they want it). The person seeks, by this manoeuvre, to get others to look after him or her and satisfy the needs he or she has not expressed. See OVERADAPTATION.

good enough (psychoanalysis) the famous phrase of Donald Winnicott (1964) who referred to the 'good enough mother'. The good enough mother is able to create a facilitating environment in which the child's needs for healthy SYMBIOSIS are met and there is enough HOLDING to contain anxiety and ward off threat. In Christopher Bollas' terms, the mother functions as a TRANSFORMATIONAL OBJECT.

Goulding, Mary transactional analyst. With her husband Robert, she founded the REDECISION SCHOOL of transactional analysis. In 1975 she received the Eric Berne Memorial Scientific Award for this work jointly with her husband.

Goulding, Robert transactional analyst. With his wife Mary, he developed redecision therapy and founded the REDECISION SCHOOL, one of the three major schools of transactional analysis (see TRANSACTIONAL ANALYSIS, SCHOOLS OF). He received the Eric Berne Memorial Scientific Award jointly with Mary in 1975 for this work.

grandiosity an exaggeration of some aspect of reality (Schiff et al., 1975). Grandiosity is the obverse of DISCOUNT-ING. Discounting involves the under-valuing or failing to take account of some aspect of reality. Each process involves the other. If I discount my own power and see myself as powerless, I also see others as having power over me (i.e. I am grandiose about their power). If I am grandiose about my power I discount the power of others.

groundedness the state of being connected to current reality. In transactional analysis terms, being in unconta-minated Adult ego-state.

grounding a procedure for increasing GROUNDEDNESS. One such procedure consists of concentrating attention alternatively on an experience of the external world and on a body experi-ence and repeating this several times.

group apparatus the functions of main-taining the group involving dealing with external aspects (telephone, fur-niture, etc.) or internal aspects such as keeping the group in order. The group leader often functions as the internal and external apparatus but Berne (1966) stresses the importance of keeping these functions clearly distinct from the function of therapist.

group dynamics the study of the psycho-logical forces that operate within a group. This has often been studied through membership of a Bion (Tavistock) group in which the facilita-tor makes few interventions and con-fines these to interpretations of the group process. This raises anxiety and leads to projection and acting out by group members, which is interpreted by the facilitator. The underlying process is therefore much nearer to psychoanalysis, on which it is based, than the much more supportive style adopted in transactional analysis groups.

group imago a mental picture of what a group is or should be like. The image of the group held by each group member. This will vary between group members

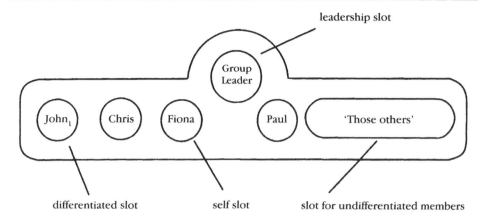

Figure 15 Partly differentiated group imago (Berne, 1963).

and may change over time. It may correspond closely to the public structure (the way the group is presented externally) but often does not. As the group develops, certain members will become significant and so be clearly differentiated while others are likely to be lumped together as 'those others' until the process of differentiation is complete. From the beginning the group leader will have a special place in the group imago. Berne's group imago diagram is often referred to as 'the submarine'. A partially differentiated group imago would be represented as shown above. See Berne (1963) and Clarkson (1992).

group therapy one or sometimes two therapists working with a group of clients. Groups provide an environment which, if well managed, can be both supportive and challenging and generate a social environment in which issues relating to the family of origin can be addressed. Clients can benefit from each other's work and this may enable them to gain insights or may trigger issues for them. Transactional analysis was usually practised as a group therapy in its early days (Berne, 1964) and with its emphasis on understanding interactions (TRANSACTIONS) it provides an excellent theoretical model for under-

standing group process. Group therapy remains important in transactional analysis although the emphasis has now shifted towards individual therapy. There tend to be two major styles of working in transactional analysis groups:

• Interactions are mainly between a client and the group leader with the group acting as a support. This was the model favoured by the Gouldings for their redecision therapy.

• Therapy is carried out within the group process with most interactions being between members, with the leader or therapist mainly intervening to control and shape the process. Many transactional analysts favour a mixture of the Goulding and process styles.

groups, stages of development Eric Berne (1963, 1966) advanced a theory of group development. Outside of transactional analysis, Tuckman and colleagues (1965, 1977) were also active in this field, identifying four stages of development occurring in small groups and calling them FORMING, STORMING, NORMING and PERFORMING. Lacousiere (1980) had suggested that there is a final stage which he called MOURNING and Tuckman and Jensen (1977) proposed the alternative name

51

of ADJOURNING and added this as a fifth stage. Clarkson (1992) has integrated Berne's group theories with this work. The following summarises her approach.

- Stage 1. Provisional GROUP IMAGO (Tuckman's *forming*). Before entering the group, potential members form a unique preconscious expectation of what the group will be like based on fantasies and previous experiences with groups.
- Stage 2. Adapted group imago (Tuckman's *storming*). The group imago is superficially modified in accordance with the member's estimate of the confronting reality. At this stage conflict and polarisation are likely to occur around interpersonal issues, thus setting up resistance to group influence and task requirements.
- Stage 3. Operative group imago (Tuckman's *norming*). The operative group imago is further modified in accordance with the member's perception of how s/he fits into the leader's imago. Ingroup feeling and cohesiveness develop, new standards evolve and new roles are adopted.
- Stage 4. Secondarily adjusted group imago (Tuckman's *performing*). The interpersonal structure of the group becomes the tool of task activities and group energy is directed into the task.
- Stage 5. Clarified group imago (Tuckman and Jensen (1977) *adjourning*, Lacousiere (1980) *mourning*). Berne identified only four stages of group development but stated that the real aim of most dynamic psychotherapy groups is to clarify the group imagos of the individual members. If the group experience has been successful in this final stage members will achieve a higher level of functioning and integration. The group has also to face its termination and deal with goodbyes and grieving.

guided fantasy (imagery) the therapist or counsellor tells a story and invites the client or clients to fantasise what is described. Discussion of the fantasies often yields important information about internal processes and fantasies can be used to evoke therapeutic change through symbolism, avoiding the interference of conscious cognitive processes. Such imaginative styles of working are valuable in contacting the Child ego-state and are particularly effective when working with the SCHIZOID PERSONALITY ADAPTATION.

gut feeling an intuitive feeling, sometimes accompanied by body sensations, thus the name. It is important that the therapist or counsellor should be open to his or her own INTUITION, which is often a useful guide and signals the activity of the LITTLE PROFESSOR, the Adult in Child ego-state A_1, but needs to be contained within the therapist's understanding of the process.

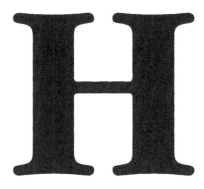

hallucination experiencing a perception (e.g. something heard or seen) in the absence of the appropriate stimulus. This indicates that the Adult ego-state is heavily contaminated, usually by Child.

hamartic script see SCRIPT, TYPES OF.

happiness one of the FOUR AUTHENTIC FEEL-INGS. A positive feeling indicating that all is going well and no changes need to be made. Its time frame is the present.

harmful intervention any intervention that reinforces script will be harmful. Examples are reinforcing a driver message or an injunction, or re-enacting within the therapy, without adequate support or protection, a trauma that led to a script decision (and so reinforcing the decision); removing or undermining a defensive system before sufficient protection is in place (e.g. confronting a driver message that is defending against a Don't Exist injunction without closing escape hatches).

here-and-now term used to emphasise the concentration on current process rather than past events or speculations about the future. The here-and-now is the province of the Adult ego-state.

hidden agenda (also referred to as covert agenda.) A set of aims, expectations, assumptions etc. that are often out of awareness but have a profound influence on the process of interpersonal transactions. The aim in the process of CONTRACTING is to make hidden agendas explicit.

historical diagnosis of ego-states the diagnosis of ego-states on the basis of knowledge of past experiences, for example a historical diagnosis of the Parent ego-state could be made if the pattern of thinking, feeling and behaving shown corresponded to an actual parental figure.

history of transactional analysis transactional analysis has a unique history among the psychotherapies. It began with Eric Berne's reaction against psychoanalysis, a discipline in which he had spent years of training. He saw it as at times too rigid and too slow to give the patient appropriate help. As a psychiatrist, particularly during his army service, he had learned the value of subtle behavioural observations. At first he used these intuitively. Later he was able to analyse them so that they could be taught. He was developing a new discipline in which behavioural and intrapsychic information could be used together so as to be mutually reinforcing. This new approach required new theory. Eric Berne read very widely and transactional analysis has been an integrative approach from its beginnings, drawing on many sources (see INTEGRATIVE THERAPY) although these were not always referenced. Berne disliked the way in which the practice of psychiatry as he had seen it tended to depower the patient. He decided that theory needs to be a shared resource between client and therapist. He therefore set out to find ways of making theory clear, vivid and accessible. Out of this fusion of the behavioural and the intrapsychic with its accessible theory and humanistic belief in the self-actualising potential of the patient, transactional analysis was born. A group of enthusiastic professionals, meeting in the San Francisco Social Psychiatry Seminars, gathered around Berne and many of the ideas of transactional analysis were worked out there.

Transactional analysis had already had an unusual history. One more event was to transform it in ways that were to have profound positive and negative consequences for the discipline. Eric Berne wrote a masterly account of his theory, *Transactional Analysis in Psychotherapy* (Berne, 1961). Regrettably, few people read it. He went on to write an account of a new aspect he was working on, which he called games theory. He included a brief and simple outline of transactional analysis theory. He called the book *Games People Play* (Berne, 1964). To his surprise it became a worldwide best seller, and transactional analysis acquired a reputation as a pop psychology. Games theory was new and what he had written about games was quickly out of date. The outline of transactional analysis theory in the book was insufficient for it to be properly

understood. *Games People Play* has contributed at least as much to the misperception of transactional analysis as it has to its reputation.

Eric Berne died in 1970 at the early age of sixty but transactional analysis has continued to develop rapidly. Its roots, like most of the major psychotherapies, are Freudian, but it has also absorbed an extraordinarily wide range of other influences, from the humanistic to the behavioural, and through the genius of Eric Berne and his co-workers and successors these have been integrated into a practical and accessible system. Because of its breadth and accessibility, it has flowed out of the usual confines of the psychotherapies into other fields such as management and education, while some see it as an important tool for independent personal development or for use in self-help groups and may approach it more as a philosophy than a therapy. Each of these fields has developed its own literature and approaches and its own way of interpreting the core literature of transactional analysis. The psychotherapeutic field has given rise to several schools of psychotherapy that, following its integrative tradition, transactional analysis has accepted into the main body of theory and practice. Transactional analysis contains examples of both assimilatory integration (in which the imported ideas are fitted within the confines of the existing system) and additive integration (in which the ideas are imported along with the matrix of theory out of which they grew). Integration on the scale that Berne undertook could not have been achieved without extensive use of the assimilatory approach with its consequent losses. One of the trends of contemporary transactional analysis is reintroducing material from other disciplines additively, especially modern psychoanalysis, to enrich the brilliantly conceived framework that Berne has left us.

histrionic personality adaptation a pattern of personality organisation characterised by ready expression of feeling and a tendency to escalate feelings when under stress. The high levels of feeling may at times interfere with clear thinking. People with this adaptation are contactful and are successful in activities that involve presenting themselves to others (e.g. acting). See PERSONALITY ADAPTATIONS, WARE SEQUENCE.

holding Donald Winnicott's term for generating a psychological environment that is perceived as safe and supportive. A parent's ability to provide this is essential for the normal development of the infant. A well-functioning family is a holding group. It is necessary to provide sufficient holding in therapy to facilitate the client in making changes, although an over-supportive environment may be counter-therapeutic. Whereas it is important to resist the client's SYMBIOTIC INVITATIONS, which seek to reinstate an archaic state of dependency, it may be appropriate at times to facilitate a relationship analogous to healthy SYMBIOSIS to enable early, unmet developmental needs to be addressed. See also CONTAINMENT, SYMBIOSIS, POTENCY.

hot potato see EPISCRIPT.

hugging embracing another person, usually by wrapping the arms round their body. The use of hugging varies between cultures and within a culture between schools of therapy. It is avoided by psychodynamic therapists and often given special emphasis by those of humanistic schools. Transactional analysis with its psychodynamic roots and strong humanistic influences falls between the two and may use hugging when, for example, highly emotional issues are dealt with however any contact between client and therapist is always contracted for.

humanistic therapy the schools of psychotherapy that emphasise the inner potential for growth and a tendency towards wholeness in human beings. The creation of the conditions favourable to growth and self-realisation, rather than dealing with pathology, is a central concern of therapy. The underlying philosophy of transactional analysis is humanistic as summarised in 'I'm OK, You're OK' but it also stresses the need to deal with the negative consequences of past experiences in order to create the conditions needed for growth and fulfilment. See PHYSIS.

hunch an intuitive idea. The therapist's hunches which usually emanate from the LITTLE PROFESSOR A_1 are important. Intuition plays a significant role in therapy but needs to be supported and checked by understanding. By following up the hunch the therapist is able to move just ahead of what he or she knows. See EMPATHY.

hunger see RECOGNITION HUNGER, STRUCTURE HUNGER, STIMULUS HUNGER.

Hurry Up one of the five DRIVERS.

hypnosis an altered state of consciousness, resembling light sleep, in which there is a raised level of suggestibility. This may be achieved by direct methods or more obliquely (e.g. Ericksonian and NLP methods). While in the trance state the client may accept suggestions that are acted on after 'waking'. Hypnotherapy is the therapeutic use of hypnosis. In transactional analysis spontaneous hypnotic processes are postulated as being involved in script formation (Clarkson, 1992) and the overall aim is to liberate the client from these influences by establishing the dominance of the Adult ego-state. It is probably for this reason that there has been relatively little interest in the therapeutic use of hypnosis by transactional analysts although it can have a positive role in facilitating the achievement of autonomy. There is currently increasing interest among transactional analysts in integrating NLP techniques. Hypnosis is sometimes sought by clients who seek change without addressing the issues of personal responsibility for actions. Its use in these circumstances is likely to be counter-therapeutic.

hypomania an energised psychological state resembling mania but less intense.

hysteric personality adaptation term formerly used for the HISTRIONIC ADAPTATION.

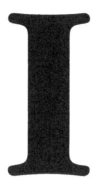

'I' statements by reformulating statements in terms of 'I . . .' a client is encouraged to take responsibility for his or her own thoughts, feelings and actions, for example 'I am feeling angry with you' rather than 'you make me angry'. This is therefore a method of confronting DISCOUNTING.

I-Thou Martin Buber's (1923, 1970) term for the authentic encounter of equals. See I'M OK, YOU'RE OK, GESTALT THERAPY, HUMANISTIC THERAPY.

ICD-10 *International Classification of Diseases,* tenth edition. A document prepared by international cooperation under the auspices of the World Health Organisation. Chapter 5 contains systems for classifying psychiatric illnesses and diagnostic criteria for the various categories. Like the DSM-IV this provides a system through which mental health professionals who have been trained in different systems can communicate by providing a common system of diagnosis. Knowledge of such a system is a requirement for qualification as a Certified Transactional Analyst.

id (psychoanalysis) an unconscious, unorganised and primitive part of the psyche, present from birth. Here are instincts arising out of the structure and functioning of the body which predate all other psychic functions. The id is characterised by PRIMARY PROCESS THINKING. The functioning of the id cannot be observed directly but must be inferred, for example, from neurotic symptoms or dreams. There are major differences between this concept and the transactional analysis concept of the Child ego-state. The contents of the Child are developed over a long period and its functioning can be inferred directly from behaviours. Its thinking, although often out of awareness, can become conscious and is not restricted to PRIMARY PROCESS, for example the Child contains decisions. In psychoanalytic terms the Child is part of the ego although responsive to early influences and drives (c.f. Fairbairn's concept of the libidinal ego). The transactional analysis concept that is closest to the id is C_0, the early Child.

identification (psychoanalysis) this term is used to describe a number of processes, all of which involve confusion regarding one's own identity and that of another person. Identity may be:

- extended into the other, making them an extension of the self;
- borrowed from the other so the self is identified with them;
- fused or confused with the other so there is no clear sense of self and other.

Primary identification occurs in infants who do not yet have a sense of the other; secondary identification occurs as a defence and the identity confusion is with someone who has been perceived as an other. Transactional analysis has not developed a unique vocabulary in this area and may employ psychoanalytic terms. See also PROJECTIVE IDENTIFICATION.

identity the unique character of the individual. Establishing an identity is an important developmental task. The RAPPROCHEMENT CRISIS is a significant stage in this process. Both the OBSESSIVE-COMPULSIVE and PASSIVE-AGGRESSIVE PERSONALITY ADAPTATIONS are associated with failures at this stage.

If It Weren't For You a GAME, initiated from the Victim position, which involves blaming someone else for failure (persecuting from a Victim position).

illustration see THERAPEUTIC OPERATIONS.

I'm OK, You're OK the healthy position in the OK CORRAL. A statement of the basic philosophical position of Transactional Analysis 'I accept myself as I am and I accept you as you are'. This does not necessarily imply approval of the other person's behaviour or of all aspects of oneself. It is about unconditional *acceptance* and *valuing* of oneself and the other person. This closely corresponds to Carl Rogers' UNCONDITIONAL POSITIVE REGARD and Martin Buber's (1923, 1970) concept of the I:THOU relationship.

I'm Only Trying To Help You a GAME initiated from the Rescuer position. This involves DISCOUNTING the abilities of the person being helped; it is driven by the Rescuer's need to Rescue rather than a measured response to the Victim's need for help.

imagery the mental pictures that clients describe symbolically represent aspects of their issues that they may find difficult to verbalise. OUTCOME FANTASIES are valuable in CONTRACTING. GUIDED FANTASY is a therapeutic technique to elicit such imagery. It facilitates contact with the Child ego-state, is particularly valuable when working with the SCHIZOID PERSONALITY ADAPTATION and also offers the opportunity to make interventions in the imagery mode (e.g. by inviting the client to imagine an image that represents or symbolises a changed life situation).

impasse an experience of being blocked or faced with an unresolvable dilemma. According to the Gouldings (Goulding and Goulding, 1979) this can take three forms which are now termed type 1, type 2 and type 3 impasses (the early literature uses the term 'degree' in place of type). Each conflict involves an internal conflict between ego-states in which Child rebels against Parent but feels unable to resolve the conflict. Resolution is ultimately achieved with the intervention of the Adult so Goulding redecision work involves contacting the Child while maintaining contact with the Adult. Mellor (1986) reformulated the Gouldings work in terms of a developmental theory, type 1 representing the latest type and type 3 the earliest. In terms of the SCRIPT APPARATUS a type 1 impasse involves counterinjunctions and a type 2 involves injunctions. The Gouldings originally formulated type 3 impasses in terms of a conflict between free (natural) Child and adapted Child; however, this involves using functional language to describe an intrapsychic process. Mellor formulates type 3 in terms of a conflict between early Parent P_0 and early Child C_0. (See Figure 16.) Since type 3 corresponds to an issue that emerged before the child had mastery of language it is often presented symbolically and reflected in body states. Impasse resolution is central to the approach of the REDECISION SCHOOL.

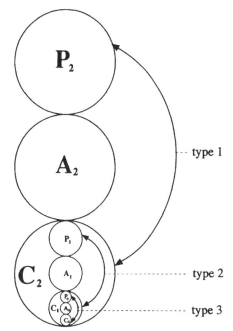

type 1

type 2

type 3

Figure 16 Types of impasses (Mellor model).

incongruity a mismatch between the content of what is said and the behaviours that accompany it, for example laughing when talking of something that is sad or frightening (the GALLOWS LAUGH) or an inconsistency between behaviours (e.g. smiling and frowning). Incongruity is an indicator of DISCOUNTING.

individuation the process of becoming a separate person, distinct from others, with one's own identity. This is a key task of DEVELOPMENT.

injunction an important negative script element held in the Child ego-state (Goulding and Goulding, 1972, 1976). An injunction is part of the SCRIPT APPARATUS and can be conceived as a negative message from the Child ego-state of an individual's parent to the person's own Child ego-state c.f. SCRIPT MATRIX, DROWNING PERSON DIAGRAM. The injunctions represent the responses of the individual's Child ego-state to unassimilated damaging material in the Child ego-state of their parent. This parent Child ego-state material affects the parent's behaviour

in ways that impact on the child but that the parent does not consciously acknowledge. The injunction forms part of the SCRIPT PROPER; that is it incorporates early decisions that are now (and perhaps always were) maladaptive. It is primary pathology rather than defence. COUNTERINJUNCTIONS are developed later and represent attempts to please the parents. When they are responded to they produce a spurious feeling of OKness as the adapted behaviour in response to the counterinjunction is felt to be pleasing the introjected parent figures in the Parent ego-state. Counterinjunctions (which make up the counterscript) therefore have a defensive function and help to neutralise the negative influence of the injunctions. Because it is the counterinjunctions that mainly determine behaviour when someone is in script, it is the mix of counterinjunctions that sets the stamp on the way in which the script is played out. Different mixes give characteristic PROCESS SCRIPTS. People who behave in the same general way when in script (who have the same process script) may have very different underlying pathology (have very different scripts proper).

Robert and Mary Goulding concluded that there are 12 main types of injunction. They labelled each of these with a phrase beginning 'Don't' because the effect of an injunction is negative, closing off potential channels of autonomous being. Their twelve injunctions are:

Don't Be (Don't Exist)
Don't Be You
Don't Be a Child
Don't Grow Up
Don't Make It
Don't Be Important (Don't Have Needs)
Don't Belong
Don't Be Close
Don't Be Well (Don't Be Sane)
Don't Think
Don't Feel (this may specify certain feelings to be excluded or may be a total ban)

Don't Do Anything (it will be wrong or dangerous)

Some transactional analysts add Don't Enjoy and Don't Trust as additional injunctions.

Verbal labels such as Don't Be Close are convenient to use and give a vivid sense of the essence of the injunction but it should not be concluded that injunctions are held only as verbal (cognitive) messages within the personality; they also involve patterns of feeling and behaving and body states. The verbal labels serve only to designate types of 'message'; each individual will have her or his own version. See MESSAGE FORMAT. However, the use of the message format does make one point clear. Injunctions are 'messages' not decisions. For the injunction to become directly active in the script the decision must be made to comply with it.

Steiner (1974) in his SCRIPT MATRIX diagram shows the injunction as being sent directly from the Child ego-state of the parent to the Child ego-state of the child. This probably describes accurately the situation in parental abuse, in which there is a gross inequality of power. In more normal parenting situations the injunction arises out of the interactions between the parent and the child and it arises out of the meanings that the child gives to the parent's behaviours. For example, the unavailability of a parent at a crucial stage in the child's development may give rise to a Don't Exist injunction but the reality that the child did not understand might have been the parent's illness. The parent did not in fact *send* the injunction. Although the injunction is primary pathology rather than defence, injunctions can be linked in defensive combinations so that one injunction defends against the other. This is called a COMPOUND DECISION (for example, I can exist as long as I don't feel).

inner child advocacy (psychoanalysis – Alice Miller) Alice Miller saw the role of the therapist as the advocate of the inner child. She derived her concept of the inner child from the transactional analysis concept of the Child ego-state and also drew on the work of John Bowlby and Karen Horney. See ADVOCACY.

insight the ability to be aware of one's own inner processes. A major aim of psychotherapy is to promote the development of insight in order to facilitate change. Transactional analysis sees insight as an Adult (A_2) function although intuition from early Adult (A_1) is also involved. The process of DECONTAMINATION by establishing boundaries between what is currently the case and what is archaic is important in this process.

Institute of Transactional Analysis the British transactional analysis organisation.

intake interview a first meeting between the client and a counsellor or psychotherapist to establish the nature of the client's problems and the suitability of the service offered to deal with them. Two important aspects to be addressed are the client's willingness to commit energy to the change process and whether he or she has sufficient available Adult ego-state to support change.

integrated Adult Berne's concept (Berne, 1961) of the final stage in the development of the Adult in which all that is of value in the Parent and Child ego-states has been assimilated and integrated within the Adult to form a single ego-state. He divides the integrated Adult into two parts: *ethos,* which contains the values and patterns of the Parent ego-state, *pathos,* which holds the Child ego-state's experience, and a central zone that he did not name. Richard Erskine has proposed the name *technos* for this part, which deals creatively with here-and-now issues. The term *logos* is also used.

integrative therapy two contrasted patterns of integration can be described as *assimilatory* and *additive*. In assimilatory integration, concepts and theories are fitted into an existing framework giving a coherent and workable system. This may be done by creating new theory. For example, Eric Berne's theory of ego-states brought together intrapsychic and interpersonal perspectives. However, integration may be purchased at the cost of extensively modifying or discarding material to achieve the fit (as in the development of LIFE POSITION theory from Melanie Klein's concepts of the PARANOID-SCHIZOID and DEPRESSIVE POSITIONS). There may also have been the loss of the unique perspective of the parent discipline and the support of its body of theory. In additive integration the transplanted material is given its own domain within the new discipline and can retain its own viewpoint and theoretical support. It is used in conjunction with the new discipline, some theoretical links being made but there is no attempt to force it into the new framework. However, this may be done at the cost of coherence or clarity. If this approach is to be successful it is necessary that there be integration at the meta-level through an overall theory that links the separate elements, giving each a place and significance within a wider framework. The worst outcome is where diverse approaches are used together without a unifying framework. Clarkson (1996) describes this as Confusion (discomfiture, embarrassment, perplexity, the action, mixture in which the distinction of the elements is lost) as opposed to Confluence (a flowing together, the junction or union of two streams). Most attempts at integration lie between these extremes. The term *integrative* is now preferred over *eclectic,* probably because it implies that something positive has been done to bring the diverse approaches together.

Transactional analysis is an integrative approach drawing on many diverse sources from behaviourism to the humanistic therapies. Eric Berne read very widely and this is clearly reflected in his thinking, although he did not always reference his sources. His successors have continued to learn from other approaches. A notable trend of recent transactional analysis, which Stewart (1996a) calls the 'psychoanalytic Renaissance', is the making of connections with other systems, in particular psychoanalysis, in a truly integrative way. An indication of the increased emphasis on integration in transactional analysis is the extension in 1990 of the criteria for the Eric Berne Memorial Award to include the integration or comparison of transactional analysis theory or practice with other therapeutic modalities. There is another sense in which the term *integrative therapy* can be used. It is a therapy whose object is to promote the integration of psychic components in the client (Erskine and Moursund, 1988; Erskine and Trautmann, 1993). Transactional analysis is also integrative in this sense. Berne (1961) envisaged the completion of psychological development as resulting in an INTEGRATED ADULT ego-state into which the valuable aspects of the former Child and Parent ego-states have become incorporated.

International Transactional Analysis Association (ITAA) the organisation, based in the United States, which seeks to coordinate transactional analysis world wide. It was the original transactional analysis organisation. All major countries now have their own national organisations, many of which are affiliated to the ITAA.

internalisation (psychoanalysis) the creation of a representation of some aspect of the external world within the mind. Internalisation is involved in the formation of the Parent ego-state. Also see INTROJECT.

internal dialogue internal communication between ego-states. This may be experienced as thoughts; for example, self-critical thoughts are probably Parent messages to Child (although if the criticisms are valid and appropriate they may be within the Adult) in response to which the Child may assent ('yes I am hopeless') or rebel ('I'll show you I'm not'). Likewise self-pitying thoughts are directed from Child to Parent. Sometimes people can hear their parents' voices in their imagination giving support, criticism or information.

internal object (psychoanalysis) see OBJECT, INTERNAL.

interpersonal between people as opposed to INTRAPSYCHIC (within the person's mind).

interposition Eric Berne (1966) described eight THERAPEUTIC OPERATIONS that he divided into two categories: interventions and interpositions. Interpositions are operations such as *illustration* in which the therapist tells a story that interposes something between the client's Adult and his or her other ego-states to prevent them slipping back.

interpretation see THERAPEUTIC OPERATIONS.

interrogation see THERAPEUTIC OPERATIONS.

intersubjectivity an awareness of a subjective self in the other person, who also has an awareness of us being aware of him or her. A theory of minds that takes into account that they are unique centres of awareness and that this awareness includes awareness of being known. Communication from an intersubjective viewpoint involves owning one's own subjective viewpoint, honouring the subjective self of the other, making an attempt intuitively to comprehend it and to communicate that it has been comprehended. Although we are all contained within a subjectivity with a unique view of the world, a fruitful dialogue is possible between our two subjectivities. This concept is inherent in the transactional analysis concept of the 'I'm OK, You're OK' LIFE POSITION. See EMPATHY.

intervention an action by the therapist designed to promote change. In Eric Berne's THERAPEUTIC OPERATIONS he distinguishes between *interventions* that impinge directly on ego-states and INTERPOSITIONS, which intervene between the client's Adult and his or her other ego-states.

intimacy close involvement with others from authentic positions, communicating needs and wants to each other openly. This is one of the six types of TIME STRUCTURING described by Eric Berne (1964). People may be intimately loving but they may also be intimately angry if they are straight and open with each other about their anger and communicate clearly from 'I'm OK, You're OK' positions. Berne (1964) defined intimacy as 'the spontaneous game-free candidness of an aware person, the liberation of the eidetically perceptive (seeing things as they are), uncorrupted Child in all its *naïveté*, living in the here and now'.

intrapsychic within the psyche or mind as opposed to INTERPERSONAL (between people).

intrauterine within the womb; i.e. before birth. It is now known that the child is aware of stimuli before birth so SCRIPT formation may occur.

introject (noun) a representation of another person taken into the internal world of the mind. The PARENT ego-state contains introjects of parent figures. Introjects function internally (e.g. in the INTERNAL DIALOGUE) in ways analogous to ways in which the original person was perceived.

introject (verb) to create an internal representation of another person. This process occurs out of awareness and without conscious intent. The person introjected will be of particular significance, such as a parent.

introvert a personality type in which there is a tendency to direct attention inward. It is often characterised by introspection, withdrawal and a tendency to become depressed. Its positive aspects include intuitiveness, creativity and performing better at tasks that require vigilance than extroverts. In Paul Ware's (1983) theory of PERSONALITY ADAPTATIONS introverts are likely to have the SCHIZOID or sometimes the OBSESSIVE-COMPULSIVE ADAPTATION. See also EXTROVERT

intuition perceiving the truth of something without reasoning or analysis. Acquiring knowledge or insight without being aware of how it has been acquired. Transactional analysis regards intuition as an early function of the mind and places it in A_1, the early Adult or Adult in Child. Because of its ability to 'suss things out' this ego-state is often referred to as the LITTLE PROFESSOR. The therapist's intuition is very important, particularly in establishing EMPATHY, because of its ability to move quickly ahead of the known. Intuition is not always reliable, however, and needs to be followed up with clear thinking from the Adult ego-state A_2.

Intuition and ego-states much of Eric Berne's earlier writings on transactional analysis appeared originally in the professional journals of psychiatry and psychoanalysis. In 1977, seven years after his death, a collection of these writings was published under the above title.

ITA INSTITUTE OF TRANSACTIONAL ANALYSIS. The UK transactional analysis organisation.

ITAA INTERNATIONAL TRANSACTIONAL ANALYSIS ASSOCIATION. The international body of transactional analysis.

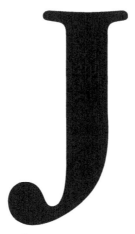

Jacobs, Alan transactional analyst. Given the Eric Berne Memorial Award in 1995 for his contributions to the theory of social applications of transactional analysis (see Jacobs, 1991). (Joint award.)

James, Muriel transactional analyst. Awarded the Eric Berne Memorial Scientific Award for developing SELF REPARENTING (James, 1974) and co-authored with Dorothy Jongeward one of the most successful introductions to transactional analysis, *Born to Win* (James and Jongeward, 1971).

jargon a derogatory term for specialised language. By implication, jargon serves to mystify and exclude those outside a small group from understanding what is being discussed. However, every speciality has unique language needs. In the development of transactional analysis the aim has been to create an open language system that can be widely shared – i.e. to avoid creating jargon. Most of its terminology draws on everyday and even colloquial expressions. To a large extent the aim of an open language system has been achieved but there has been a cost. Inappropriate meanings are carried over from the everyday use of words; for example, a GAME in transactional analysis is unlike the everyday concept of a 'game'. Also the use of familiar words in place of technicalities sometimes leads to transactional analysis being misperceived as theoretically lightweight. See LANGUAGE OF TRANSACTIONAL ANALYSIS.

Joines, Vann received the Eric Berne Memorial Award in Transactional Analysis (joint award) in 1994 for his work on using redecision therapy with different personality adaptations (Joines, 1986) and diagnosis and treatment planning using a transactional analysis framework (Joines, 1988). He is joint author (with Ian Stewart) of a popular introduction to transactional analysis (*TA Today*, Stewart and Joines, 1987).

Jung, Carl analyst. Jung was at first closely associated with Freud but later left psychoanalysis to found his own school which he called 'analytical psychology'. Jung's thought ranged widely and he was deeply interested in myth and symbolism. He aimed to create a system that was more open and broader than Freud's psychoanalysis but his approach lacks Freud's clarity and consistency. Eric Berne trained as a psychoanalyst so the underlying assumptions of transactional analysis tend to have Freudian roots but Jung's ideas had an influence on his thinking on script. For the integration of Jungian ideas into transactional analysis, see Merlin (1977).

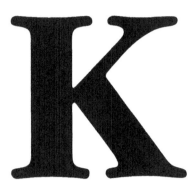

Kahler, Taibi transactional analyst who has made major contributions to theory. He received the Eric Berne Memorial Scientific Award in 1977 for his work on the MINISCRIPT and the five DRIVERS (Kahler and Capers, 1974). Taibi Kahler has also developed Paul Ware's concept of PERSONALITY ADAPTATION in his process therapy approach.

Karpman, Stephen transactional analyst. He was awarded the Eric Berne Memorial Scientific Award twice, in 1972, for his work on the DRAMA TRIANGLE (Karpman, 1968 – the drama triangle is sometimes referred to as the Karpman Triangle), and again in 1979 for his work on OPTIONS (Karpman, 1971).

Kick Me game initiated from the Victim position and inviting persecution.

This reinforces the initiator's belief that he or she is no good but also enables the Victim to get negative strokes and thus know that he or she exists.

Klein, Melanie Austrian-born psychoanalyst. She came to England from Berlin (where she had been analysed by FERENCZI) in 1927 and became the centre of the British School out of which grew the OBJECT RELATIONS approach. She worked mainly with children and developed a highly original theoretical approach stressing the importance of very early experiences and conflicts. Some of her ideas have been influential in the development of transactional analysis (e.g. she originated the concept of the LIFE POSITION).

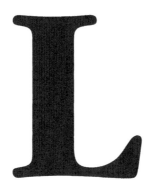

language of transactional analysis
transactional analysis has developed its
own distinctive language. As one of the
aims of the discipline is maximum accessibility this largely uses everyday words
although it gives them a distinctive
meaning. This makes the language less
threatening but the technical meaning,
although it may resemble the everyday
one, is never the same (for example a
Bernian game differs profoundly from
football). This problem is not confined
to transactional analysis: physicists give
the word energy a meaning which
resembles but differs significantly from
everyday usage. However the decision
of transactional analysis to draw most of
its vocabulary from everyday speech has
brought disadvantages. In addition to
the differences in meaning and usage,
the use of commonplace terms or even
slang (e.g. racket, gimmick) to express
technical meanings may lead to transactional analysis being misperceived as
'light weight'. See JARGON.

**Layman's Guide to Psychiatry and
Psychoanalysis** Eric Berne's first
book. See *A Layman's Guide*.

laughter Berne (1972) identified six
types of laughter of which three are
SCRIPT SIGNS and three healthy.

1. The scripty laugh from negative Parent in Child (P_1, often called the witch
mother or the ogre father) leading
someone into derision and defeat.
2. The Adult's chuckle of rueful humour
at achieving a limited insight into his
or her self-destructive behaviour
from which he or she has yet to
release him- or herself. This is the GAL-
LOWS LAUGH.
3. The Child's laugh when he is about
to pull a fast one (but is likely to end
up a Victim). This is the gamy laugh.
4. The Parent's laugh at the Child's
struggle to succeed. This is essentially
benevolent and helpful but also may
be patronising. This is the grandad
or Santa Claus laugh.
5. A laugh that is much more hearty and
meaningful and signifies full insight
by the Adult into how she or he has
been 'conned' by his or her own Parent and Child. This is the laugh of
insight.
6. The Child's laugh of sheer fun and
enjoyment. This is the spontaneous
laugh of healthy people.

Levin, Pamela transactional analyst.
Received the Eric Berne Memorial
Scientific Award in 1984 for her work
on developmental cycles (Levin, 1982,
1988). She offers the most complete
account of child development within
transactional analysis theory, drawing
on Freud, Mahler, Erikson and her
own research. She draws attention to
the transferential reactivation of devel-

opmental issues by life events, for example activation of oral (first year) issues often follows a new beginning. She also suggests that recycling though all the stages of child development continue throughout the life cycle and she identifies ages at which specific stage issues are likely to become salient.

leadership hunger Berne (1966) the need of a group for a leader to provide time structuring. This is a derivative of STRUCTURE HUNGER.

libido (psychoanalysis) originally a form of mental energy deriving from the ID (from the instinctual level of the psyche) and associated with sexuality. Later Freud used it as a more general term for mental energy, for example the EGO was assumed to possess ego-libido. In later psychoanalytic instinct theory libido is the energy of the life instinct (love). Berne uses the term *cathexis* or *energy* but postulates that it can exist in three states; bound, unbound and free. See ENERGY. The opposite of libido, the energy of the death instinct (Thanatos) is a concept which is little used. However it has been given the name Mortido. An alternative name which is sometimes used is Destrudo.

life events the individual's life will have been shaped by life events, each of which may have encouraged or reinforced script beliefs and led to early decisions. The early stages of therapy usually include exploration of significant past life events. These may be both the cause and the result of scripting since, as script is formed, it influences subsequent events. Events occurring during therapy are often closely related to script issues being addressed and may constitute manifestations of GAMES or ACTING OUT.

life positions also known as existential positions or basic positions (Berne, 1962, 1966, 1972). Each represents an outlook on life that has a profound effect on the way the world is construed and life is lived. There are four life positions:

1. 'I'm OK, you're OK' (I+U+). 'I accept myself unconditionally as I am and I accept you unconditionally as you are.' This is the healthy position enabling the person to be autonomous and to form relationships that are balanced and rewarding. 'You're OK' does not mean that I approve of everything that you do but that I unconditionally accept your value as a person. c.f. UNCONDITIONAL POSITIVE REGARD.
2. 'I'm not OK, you're OK' (I−U+). Individuals in this position constantly look to others for approval, undervalue themselves and are subject to depression.
3. I'm OK, you're not OK (I+U−). The person in this position is critical and mistrustful of others but lacks insight into what they are doing. This is characteristic of paranoid disorders although many people enter this state from time to time.
4. I'm not OK, you're not OK (I−U−). This is a despairing position that often underlies serious psychological disorders.

All four positions occur from time to time in relatively healthy ('normal') people but they are quickly able to move back into the healthy position. It is fixedness in one of the unhealthy positions that constitutes a problem The concept was originated by Melanie KLEIN. See also OK CORRAL, DEPRESSIVE POSITION, PARANOID-SCHIZOID POSITION.

life script the unconscious life plan derived from early experiences that governs the way life is lived out. Usually referred to simply as SCRIPT.

literature of transactional analysis the main journal of transactional analysis is the *Transactional Analysis Journal* (TAJ) published by the International Transactional Analysis Association. This was preceded by an earlier publication, the *Transactional Analysis Bulletin* (TAB). In addition, most national associations publish their own journals. That of the British organisation (the Institute of Transactional Analysis) is the *ITA News*. Because of the wide area of application of transactional analysis and the variety of levels at which it can be addressed, books on transactional analysis cover a wide range, from popularisation to technically advanced works. Some books attempt to cover this wide range. Berne's last book, *What Do You Say After You Say Hello?* might be seen as doing this. *Games People Play* became a best seller by accident and was not designed as a popular book. His *Principles of Group Practice* is unequivocally technical. The best exposition of transactional analysis theory is also the first, Berne's *Transactional Analysis in Psychotherapy*. Some popularisations do a good job of conveying the basics of the approach but others are at times inaccurate, or oversimplified and have contributed to the misunderstanding (and perhaps misuse) of transactional analysis ideas. A brief reading list is included in Appendix 1 to provide some guidance to anyone making his or her first contact with the literature. In order to keep it brief it was necessary to leave out many meritorious books, so the omission of any book does not indicate criticism.

Little Professor the Adult in Child A_1. In this subdivision of the Child ego-state we find early, non-logical intuitive thinking patterns that enable the individual to get answers quickly with minimum background information – to be 'smart' rather than 'intelligent'. This type of thinking is very valuable provided logical (A_2) thinking is also used alongside it to provide checks.

loss the object relations theorist John Bowlby (1969) drew attention to the importance of attachments to other people, stemming from the attachment of a child to her or his parents. This attachment extends to attachment to material objects, places, activities etc. Loss of something to which one is attached, be it a friend or a toy, brings grief and initiates a process of mourning. Issues of loss are often the precipitating factors bringing people into therapy. Often a loss will activate unresolved grief remaining from earlier losses. Therapy itself may re-enact loss (for example, when the therapist goes away or when the therapy comes to an end). See MOURNING.

low self-esteem the person with low self-esteem is in the 'I'm not OK, you're OK' LIFE POSITION. Early experiences will have led to negative script beliefs and INJUNCTIONS such as Don't Exist, Don't Be You and Don't Be Important are likely to be present. Among transactional analysts, Jean Illesley Clarke (1978) has worked extensively on the issue of self-esteem.

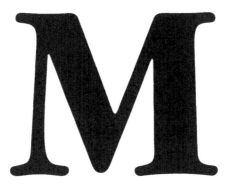

magical Parent the Parent in the Child ego-state. See P_1.

magical thinking young children do not distinguish clearly between thought and action and so may believe that their thoughts (for example, hostile feelings towards their parents) can directly affect others. A child may feel responsible for a relative's death or illness or the conflict between his or her parents. Children may also believe that the world may be changed in some way by wishing it to be different, a theme of many fairy stories. This style of thinking is referred to as magical thinking and is particularly characteristic of the five year old, thus the name MAGICAL PARENT for the early version of the Parent ego-state P_1. See also OMNIPOTENCE.

maladaptive maladaptive patterns of thinking, feeling or behaviour are not appropriate to current reality although they may have been appropriate at some time in the past.

mania a highly energised psychological state in which the client may talk constantly, sleep very little and have grandiose beliefs about his or her abilities.

manic-depressive a disorder in which there are major mood swings between a highly excited manic phase and deep

depression; the condition in which the mood swings are not so severe is known as cyclothymia. Loomis and Landsman (1980) have advanced a theory of the manic-depressive structure and a treatment approach based on the concept of ego-state splitting.

marshmallows insincere positive strokes. The practice of giving these strokes is referred to as 'throwing marshmallows'.

marathon extended group therapy lasting from one to several days. This maximises processes and provides a safe space in which intensive work can be done.

Martian we have all been trained to see social interactions in particular ways. The Martian view is the totally objective view of someone who comes from outside our culture. Children have this view before they are indoctrinated into the rules of society. Transactional analysis encourages us to take a Martian view, to stand back and see things as they are actually occurring and also to 'speak Martian', to say what we see and what we feel.

McNeel, John received the Eric Berne Memorial Award in Transactional Analysis in 1994 for his work on the PARENT INTERVIEW (McNeel, 1976).

meaning the significance given to experience in the mind, the way it is related to other experiences, value systems, beliefs, etc. According to transactional analysis, each individual creates a FRAME OF REFERENCE (FOR) that incorporates his or her system of meanings at all levels, not just conscious knowledge and beliefs (Schiff et al., 1975). All incoming experience is processed using the FOR. Since early decisions and beliefs that have not been updated will be incorporated in the FOR it is the repository of SCRIPT. Whenever an early decision or belief that is no longer valid is used to process current experience, this can be done only if some aspects of current reality are DISCOUNTED (because if they were accounted the belief or decision would have to be changed). Responding within script therefore always involves discounting. Stewart and Joines (1987) define script as that part of the FOR that involves discounting.

medical model the term 'medical model' was used by Eric Berne (1971) to signify a model of psychological treatment that stresses dealing with causes rather than symptoms and aims to bring about CURE. Berne (1971) made the analogy with a patient with a splinter in his toe; this would lead to all sorts of secondary problems e.g postural problems, but dealing with these would not effect CURE. The cure could only be effected by identifying that the problems stemmed from the splinter and removing it. The term 'medical model' is frequently used today to describe the approach in psychiatry that sees psychological problems as mainly deriving from disturbances in brain biochemistry and consequently lays heavy stress on the use of drugs.

medication the use of drugs that affect feelings and thought processes (psychotropic drugs). Medication is important in the management of acute mental illness but may be an obstacle to therapy by making thoughts and feelings less available to the client (for example, they may make the Child less accessible and the Adult less active).

Mellor, Ken Australian transactional analyst. Worked for a time within the Cathexis movement and is one of the authors of the Cathexis reader (Schiff et al., 1975). With Eric Sigmund, was jointly awarded an Eric Berne Memorial Scientific Award in 1980 for his work on discounting and redefining (Mellor and Sigmund, 1975). Made a contribution to redecision theory by proposing a developmental model of the three impasses (see REDECISION). With his wife, Elizabeth, he became deeply interested in eastern mysticism and has developed an original system of therapy incorporating meditation.

memory memories can be of many kinds, for example memories of facts, memories of feelings, memories of experiences, memories of sequences of events. Ego-states are made up of total memories of past life experiences. These memories include ways of thinking, feeling and behaving and experiencing. For example, the Child ego-state contains many such memories of childhood; it is more accurate to talk about Child ego-states than the Child ego-state, although that is common usage. When Child is contacted it is usually at a particular point – it is one phase of childhood that is being contacted. The Parent ego-state is likewise made up of memories of significant others, the parents and other people who were significant in childhood.

mental health health is to be seen positively, it is not just the absence of disease. In Eric Berne's (1961) original formulation it would involve the achievement of INTEGRATED ADULT functioning in which the Adult has been able to integrate and have available for use the valuable material from the Child and Parent ego-states but is no longer influenced by the negative material. This would mean that the individual would be truly autonomous. Berne (1957, 1972) writes of a drive towards wholeness and fulfilment that he calls PHYSIS and represents by an upward arrow passing through all three ego-states (thus formulating the principles of humanistic therapy in drive terms). Health must also involve the free flow of physis.

mental illness a state of prolonged psychological distress or a state in which the community does not accept behaviours. Thomas Szasz (1961) pointed out the very large social component in mental illness. The term isolates the problem within the client but it exists not only within the client but also within his or her relationships, including those with the external society. Pressures of the society or the family or group in which the client lives may make it very difficult for them not to experience distress or behave in ways that are not acceptable to others. Transactional analysis starts from the position 'I'm OK, You're OK', that is 'I accept you as you are and I accept myself as I am, although I may not accept what you are doing'. Transactional analysts do not tell people what is wrong with them but invite them to make a contract for change; this contract must be acceptable to both the client and the therapist. To make such a contract the client must have functional Adult available. Transactional analysis takes the position that most people including children have this and that it is important to empower clients to use their Adult resources and not to rescue them when this would be inappropriate because they have the resources to help themselves. In some cases, such as psychosis, Adult is not available and a contractual approach is not appropriate while the client remains in this situation. This raises complex ethical issues for the therapist. These gave rise to the controversy regarding the Schiffs' work with schizophrenics. See also CURE.

mental organs see PSYCHIC ORGANS.

message format transactional analysts frequently refer to 'messages' influencing the client and may use imagery such as 'the Parent whispering in the Child's ear' or 'Parent tapes playing in the head'. Verbal labels in message format such as a Don't Be Close injunction or a Try Hard driver are convenient to use and give a vivid sense of the essence of the concept and how it functions intrapsychically, but it should not be concluded that they imply that the intrapsychic features which they name exist solely as verbal messages held within the personality. Powerful injunctions (such as Don't Exist) are often received before the child is capable of speech. The injunction and other script elements involve cognitive (thoughts), affective (feelings), behavioural and physical (body states) components. The message format for representing intrapsychic elements is characteristic of the metaphor used in transactional analysis; it is one of the features that give it its vividness, accessibility, precision and brevity. However, when not understood it can lead to transactional analysis being misperceived as a simplistic approach. By contrast, the object relations theorist Wilfred Bion aimed to create a terminology that opened up a space into which the individual's own, experientially derived meaning might enter. He wrote: 'the advantage of employing a sign . . . is that it at least indicates that the reader's comprehension of my meaning should contain an element that will remain unsatisfied until he meets the appropriate realisation'. There is the risk that the metaphor of transactional analysis leads to the meaning being perceived as clearer than it really is; however, the ability to identify and specify injunctions, for example, opens up possibilities for treatment planning that would not be available without the insights of transactional analysis and the precision of its language.

methodology of transactional analysis transactional analysis seeks links between observable behaviours and intrapsychic states. It is thus able to maintain a position that is simultaneously behaviourist and intrapsychically analytic. This dual stance is particularly valuable in dealing with interactions (TRANSACTIONS) between individuals. The person is thus studied both as an individual and as a social unit in communication with others, yielding a two-person perspective on psychology.

miniscript a process in which a section of script process is played though in a short period of time (seconds or minutes). The process involves responding to an external or internal stressor by going into DRIVER BEHAVIOUR from an ADAPTED CHILD position. The driver is a defensive manoeuvre so no emotion is felt while it functions. When it fails to maintain equilibrium the person

moves into one of three positions:

1. Stopper. Here the LIFE POSITION is I–U+ and the person is responding to the negative message of an INJUNCTION from adapted Child and experiencing RACKET FEELINGS such as guilt, hurt, worry, embarrassment or confusion.
2. Blamer. Here the life position is I+U– and rackets such as blameful, triumphant, spiteful, blameless or furious are operated from a spiteful adapted Child or negative controlling Parent position.
3. Despairer. Here the life position is I–U–, the ego-state is negative adapted Child and typical rackets are worthless, unwanted, hopeless, cornered, unloved, futile.

Movement can occur between these positions (a common sequence is stopper, despairer, blamer). Eventually there is a return to a driver and a new sequence begins. There is a similarity between the concepts of miniscript and GAMES, which both include time-limited sequences involving rackets that advance the script.

mirroring showing in one's behaviour awareness and responsiveness to the

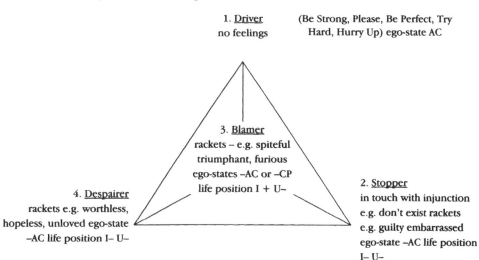

1. <u>Driver</u>
no feelings

(Be Strong, Please, Be Perfect, Try Hard, Hurry Up) ego-state AC

3. <u>Blamer</u>
rackets – e.g. spiteful
triumphant, furious
ego-states –AC or –CP
life position I + U–

2. <u>Stopper</u>
in touch with injunction
e.g. don't exist rackets
e.g. guilty embarrassed
ego-state –AC life position
I– U–

4. <u>Despairer</u>
rackets e.g. worthless,
hopeless, unloved ego-state
–AC life position I– U–

Figure 17 Miniscript (Kahler and Capers, 1974).

client and his or her experiences so that they are able to become aware of themselves through the therapist. This is a way of giving PERMISSIONS, to exist, to feel and to be oneself.

missed sessions the business contract (see CONTRACT) needs to deal with what will happen if the Client misses a session. Missing or being late for sessions is a common way in which Clients show resistance to therapy and is very often a move to invite the therapist into a GAME.

model (noun) A representation of a system or process in other terms, for example the ego-state model of the personality. This can be expressed diagrammatically or verbally and is an effective way of displaying information about the structure and function of the ego. A model is a metaphor designed to be isomorphous with some aspect of reality (it provides a 'map' of some aspect or aspects of experience).

Psychological disturbances (which will often be linked to physiological disturbances) can be explained in terms of three models (Clarkson, 1992). In the *confusion model* there is interference in the functioning of the Adult ego-state in an integrated way with other ego-states. This can be represented as CONTAMINA-TION. In the *conflict model* there is conflict between ego-states as represented in the IMPASSE concept of REDECISION therapy. The *deficit model* describes how disturbances result from developmental deficits (missed experiences needed for development) and inadequate parenting for extended periods at the time of trauma. Another way of representing these ideas is Lee's (1988b) concept of the PRIMAL WOUND.

model (verb) To give a message, for example a permission, through behaviour. A parent might give a permission to express sadness to a child by showing his own sadness, thus modelling the permission 'it is OK to be sad'.

Moiso, Carlo received the Eric Berne Memorial Award in Transactional Analysis in 1987 for his work on ego-states and transference (Moiso, 1985).

mortido (psychoanalysis) the energy associated with the death instinct; c.f. LIBIDO referred to by Berne (1957). There is no corresponding concept in transactional analysis ENERGY theory although the concept of the script PAY-OFF bears some resemblance to Freud's thinking about the death instinct.

mother a female parent or anyone who fulfils the main role in providing the care and support needed by the developing child (sets up and maintains healthy SYMBIOSIS). Good mothering can be given by people who are not biologically related to the child (or even not female).

motivation that which tends to bring about action. An important aspect is the meaning attached to the action by the individual; this will depend on the content of their FRAME OF REFERENCE. Out of awareness factors are often involved in motivation so that people find themselves unwilling to do the things they 'ought' to do (that is, the things their Parent ego-state tells them to do) but find themselves doing things they think they ought not to do (things that may be EGO DYSTONIC with Adult or Parent). Transactional analysis explains this in terms of the distribution of energy across ego-states. See ENERGY.

mourning the process of letting go of an attachment (usually an attachment to a person) on separation, death etc. Kubler-Ross (1969) identified a five-stage sequence: denial, anger, bargaining, depression and acceptance. Lacousiere identified mourning as a final stage in group development in which the group focuses on its termination. See GROUPS, STAGES OF DEVELOPMENT.

MPD multiple personality disorder. A dissociative disorder in which the personality is split into a number of distinctive sub-personalities that manifest more or less independently. See DISSOCIATION.

mutuality a mode of interaction between two people in which there is mutual respect and each takes account of the other's unique view of the world. It will involve each maintaining an 'I'm OK, You're OK' position, being open (transactional analysis – 'talking MARTIAN'; Rogers – 'being congruent') and being insightful and empathic. The counsellor or therapist needs to offer mutuality and create an environment where it is safe; the client may need time to check this out. Sometimes the achievement of full mutuality is an indicator that therapy is complete. See INTERSUBJECTIVITY.

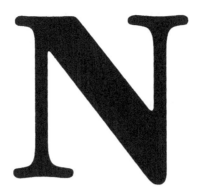

narcissism investment of psychological energy (cathexis) in the self. This may be positive and helpful (for example, healthy self-respect). Over-valuation of the self is a defence, often against the trauma of early loss of relationship. Psychoanalysts distinguish between *primary narcissism*, the baby's love of self that precedes loving others, and *secondary narcissism* that involves INTROJECTING and identifying with an OBJECT. The child needs positive responses to nurture and sustain the self; these can be termed *narcissistic needs* and might be represented in transactional analysis terms as adequate and appropriate STROKES. Rejecting and abusive behaviour towards the child inflicts a *narcissistic wound* and would be likely to result in a Don't Exist INJUNCTION.

natural Child (also written Natural Child) when someone reacts from a spontaneous and open Child position, in touch with emotions and reacting to the moment with enthusiasm and energy, we describe him or her as being in the natural Child ego-state. Although such a person will be responsive to others he or she will be in touch with his or her own needs and wants and will seek openly to satisfy them. This is to be contrasted with the adapted Child in which behaviour is constrained by adaptation to the (assumed) needs and wishes of others as it had been in childhood to the parents. This is a functional concept, i.e. it describes the outward (behavioural) manifestation of an ego-state. See FUNCTIONAL EGO-STATES.

need something that is necessary for normal healthy functioning. This includes not only physical needs such as food and warmth but also psychological needs. Transactional analysis stresses the importance of RECOGNITION HUNGER, which is satisfied through STROKING, and STRUCTURE HUNGER, which signifies a need for TIME STRUCTURING.

negative stroke a STROKE is an act of recognition from another person. Stroking is required to maintain psychological health. Berne (1964) described strokes as units of social action. Strokes can take many forms, verbal and non-verbal, negative and positive. A negative stroke is hostile, rejecting, undermining or critical, for example a disparaging remark. However, the verbal or non-verbal act is directed towards the person and therefore involves recognising their existence. Negative strokes are sometimes sought for this reason. Many children find that negative strokes are easier to elicit from their parents than positive ones and learn to do this to avoid being stroke deprived. This may become the basis of a lifelong pattern of seeking negative strokes. See STROKE QUOTIENT.

neopsyche Berne (1961) postulated three psychic organs that manifested themselves phenomenologically as three ego-states. The neopsyche is the psychic organ that manifests as the Adult ego-state. He wrote 'The methodological problems involved in moving from organs to phenomena to substantives are not relevant to practical applications.' Transactional analysts have followed this precept and tend to use the term *ego-state* in a way that is inclusive of all three concepts. See ARCHEOPSYCHE, EXTEROPSYCHE.

neurolinguistic programming (commonly abbreviated NLP) is a form of cognitive therapy originated by Richard Bandler and John Grinder (1975). It arose from their work in the 1960s in which they studied the practice of other therapists such as Virginia Satir, Fritz Perls and Milton Erickson. It operates by identifying and isolating the linguistic strategies that are observed to bring about change in clients. Neurolinguistic programming has now integrated into its theory the cybernetic concepts of feedback and feed-forward and the fractal model of language and aims to make small changes that propagate throughout an individual's conceptual model of his or her world. Neurolinguistic programming is a meta model (a model of how the client models his or her world) and pays attention to what is said in order to understand how the client recorded his or her memories (visually, auditorily or kinesthetically and so forth) and how this relates to his or her behaviours. As it is based on working with observable behaviours, NLP has a high computability with transactional analysis as both approaches involve linking behaviours with intrapsychic states.

neurosis originally psychoneurosis. A psychological disturbance that causes distress but where the client has insight and acknowledges the problem as his or hers. This contrasts with personality disorders (character disorders), in which the problem is usually attributed to others (a loss of contact with social reality), and psychosis, in which there is a loss of contact with many aspects of consensual reality resulting in major disturbances of thinking, feeling and behaviour. The term neurosis is now less often used and is not included in DSM-IV. Since the central characteristic of neurosis is that the client has insight and is prepared to acknowledge problems, it seems unreasonable that this should be named as a form of pathology.

NIGYYSOB 'Now I've Got You, You Son Of A Bitch.' Persecutory game initiated from a Victim position. Bernian GAMES describe recognisable sequences of behavioural interactions that are widely observable. In the early development of games theory there was concentration on the specific behavioural pattern and this resulted in the naming of numerous games, usually with colloquial, snappy titles. Later it was realised that these fall into a relatively small number of general patterns. Transactional analysts now tend to concentrate on a small number of game types that are usually referred to by the name of the best known example. NIGYYSOB is a typical Persecutor game that involves a CON of a request for assistance responded to by GIMMICKY helpfulness. Having initiated from a Victim position, the initiator of the game now switches to Persecutor (you have not helped me properly so I am going to get you). Games involve two (occasionally more) people in unauthentic roles (both are playing a game), so in a behavioural interaction two games are going on. NIGYYSOB is likely to be matched by a Victim game such as I'm Only Trying to Help You, which is initiated from a Rescuer position and ends up in Victim. See DRAMA TRIANGLE.

NLP see NEUROLINGUISTIC PROGRAMMING

non-directive Following the client and being purely reflective. Rogers originally named his approach to counselling 'non-directive' but changed it later to 'client centred' and most Rogerians now prefer the term 'person centred' to acknowledge the equality of the two people who engage in the process. Rogers' thinking has had an influence on many schools of psychotherapy, including transactional analysis, by raising awareness of the importance of empowering the client and acknowledging the client's unique perspective. Transactional analysis recognises the importance of facilitating the client on his or her journey rather than taking the client along, but believes that theory provides a map and a therapist who can read the map and share its insights with the client can ensure a quicker and safer journey.

non-verbal communication information about states of mind, feelings etc. signalled by non-verbal means such as paralinguistics (tone of voice, speech rhythms), facial expression, eye contact, body posture and movement patterns. Transactional analysts are trained to observe such behaviours carefully as they provide much information on EGO-STATES. Incongruence between verbal and non-verbal communication indicates ULTERIOR TRANSACTIONS.

normal behaviour behaviour viewed within a particular culture as healthy, well adjusted and socially acceptable. There are wide variations between cul-

tures in what is considered normal and this changes over time. Normal is also used in the sense of what commonly occurs even if it is not culturally endorsed as in 'it is normal to lose your temper occasionally'. Clients often become concerned as to whether their behaviour is normal. They are usually responding to critical messages from their Parent ego-state and may require PERMISSIONS from the therapist. There is usually a need for clear Adult information about what is possible and acceptable in their culture. This may lead to a change in their FRAME OF REFERENCE.

normal dependency children lack the personal resources to meet many of their needs for themselves so are dependent on their parents. This dependency becomes less as they mature until they are capable of becoming fully autonomous individuals. If their dependency is appropriate to their developmental stage (they are allowed and encouraged to be as autonomous as is safe and healthy), they are in a state of normal dependency. This will be characterised by HEALTHY SYMBIOSIS (that is the parent or caregiver provides for those needs that the development of the child's EGO-STATES do not yet make it possible for them to supply for themselves but allow the child to have as much AUTONOMY as they can sustain). Unhealthy dependency is usually developed in response to parents' emotional needs and may become a lifelong pattern (SECOND-ORDER SYMBIOSIS).

normative concerning norms and standards. These are often valuable, for example standards of professional practice, but can be oppressive. The contractual process in transactional analysis facilitates the separation of the necessary standard from the norm that discounts the value and the uniqueness of the client. See CONTRACT.

norming the establishment of norms and standards. Tuckman (1965) recognised a number of distinct stages in the forming of a group and Clarkson (1992) has integrated his ideas with Berne's (1963) theories. In Tuckman's norming stage the group becomes pre-occupied with establishing how things should be done. See GROUPS, STAGES OF DEVELOPMENT.

nursing triad a term originated by the object relations theorist Donald Winnicott for the child being cared for by the mother who in her turn is cared for by the father. Using the Schiff

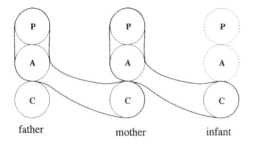

father   mother   infant

Figure 18 Nursing triad (healthy first-order symbiosis – no discounting) (Schiff et al., 1975). Winnicott's concept of the nursing triad as a symbiosis diagram.

healthy SYMBIOSIS diagram it can be represented as in Figure 18.

An analogous relationship may exist between client, therapist and supervisor.

nurturing Parent (often written Nurturing Parent) When someone is behaving in a caring and supportive way towards others from a Parent position, we describe them as being in the nurturant Parent ego-state. This is a functional concept, that is, it describes the outward (behavioural) manifestation of an ego-state. See FUNCTIONAL EGO- STATES.

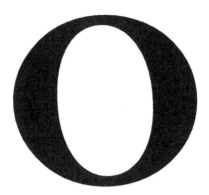

object (psychoanalysis) this word has a meaning that is different from its everyday usage. It means not a material thing but something to which a subject relates. In practice this usually means a person, a part of a person (e.g. the mother's breast) or something that represents a person. See also TRANSITIONAL OBJECT, TRANSFORMATIONAL OBJECT.

object constancy (Kleinian psychoanalysis) the ability to accept the ambivalence of others (the child's ability to recognise at the deepest level that the mother who frustrates is also the mother who nurtures). See also PARANOID-SCHIZOID POSITION, OBJECT PERMANENCE.

object, internal (psychoanalysis) an internal representation of an external object (e.g. person) that one relates to as if it were an external object. The representations of the parents within the Parent ego-state can be regarded as internal objects. This concept is central to the thinking of the OBJECT RELATIONS SCHOOL, which has had a significant influence on transactional analysis.

object permanence (Piaget) the stage in child development where the child shows signs of recognising the continuing existence of an object when it is not visible.

object relations school (psychoanalysis) a therapeutic approach that stresses the psychological importance of relationship to both external and internal OBJECTS. This contrasts with classical Freudian drive theory, which focused on the need to reduce internal tension caused by instinctual demands emerging from the ID. Object relations theory was an influence on transactional analysis; the Parent ego-state is in essence a group of internal objects (introjected parent figures). Recent developments in transactional analysis have been characterised by a renewed interest in psychoanalysis, in particular object relations and self psychology. Stewart (1996a) refers to this as 'the psychoanalytic renaissance'.

obsessive-compulsive personality adaptation an adaptation (that is a characteristic way of reacting compatible with normal life) which shows some of the features of obsessive-compulsive disorder (Ware, 1983). It is characterised by a methodical and orderly approach and a need to get things right and gain approval. The person has a need for information and seeks to stay in control by understanding and thinking and has difficulty accessing feeling. He or she also has difficulty in making decisions and changing behaviour patterns. The underlying psychological issue is the lack of an emotionally safe world in childhood. The major driver is Be Perfect. This pattern is also referred to as the Workaholic. See also PERSONALITY ADAPTATION.

Oedipus complex (psychoanalysis) the wish (usually out of awareness) to form a strong bond with the parent of the opposite sex and to displace or get rid of the parent of the same sex. Freud places the peak age for this at three to five as the child's sense of sexual identity is emerging. If it is not resolved it will have long-term effects. Melanie Klein held that the Oedipus complex could emerge in the first year of life. Unresolved oedipal issues are often involved in the development of the histrionic PERSONALITY ADAPTATION. The term originally applied only to males, the female equivalent being the Electra complex. The term Oedipus complex is now used for both sexes.

oedipal stage (psychoanalysis) in Freud's theory of psychosexual development, the stage at which the child becomes aware of their gender identity and seeks a special or exclusive relationship with the parent of the opposite sex. See OEDIPUS COMPLEX.

ogre the negative aspect of P_1, the Parent in Child. Also known as the witch Parent and the pig Parent.

OK corral a way of presenting Berne's four LIFE POSITIONS diagrammatically developed by Ernst (1971). An abbreviated notation is often used for the life positions. I+ stands for 'I'm OK' and U+ for 'you're OK', similarly I– and U– for the not-OK viewpoints. Each of the four quadrants also contains the process that arises from the life position. For example, for the 'I'm OK, you're not OK' quadrant the process is 'get rid of'. 'You are the problem, if I get rid of you I solve my problem!' Each

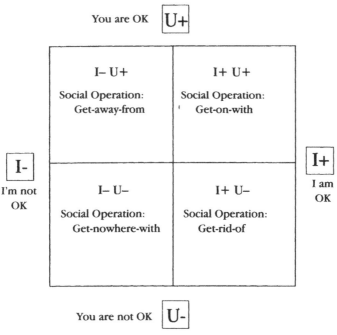

The OK Corral: Grid For What's Happening

Figure 19 OK corral (Ernst, 1971).

quadrant also has a name for the state that it represents. The 'I'm not OK, You're not OK' is the futility (also called despairing or schizoid) position. We all visit all the quadrants from time to time but everyone has a favoured life position in which they spend most of their time. We move through the quadrants over the short term as our mood changes and over the long term as we change because of life experience or therapy. It is not possible to move directly from the paranoid to the healthy position. This change involves visiting the depressive (I–U+) and perhaps also the futility (I–U–) positions. This corresponds to Melanie Klein's view of the depressive position as representing an advance in functioning over the paranoid-schizoid position (achievement of OBJECT CONSTANCY). See LIFE POSITIONS, PARANOID-SCHIZOID POSITION, DEPRESSIVE POSITION.

OKness the state of being in an 'I'm OK, You're OK' LIFE POSITION. See 'I'M OK, YOU'RE OK', OK CORRAL, OPENNESS.

omnipotence belief in being all-powerful. This is probably normal in early infancy but the child learns the limits of his or her powers through repeated experiences of frustration. In the adult, the belief that events conform, or should conform, to their wishes is dysfunctional. Belief in the omnipotence of thought (that thought can directly affect others or the external world) underlies MAGICAL THINKING and may explain why wishes can evoke as much guilt as actions.

openness the state of being direct, non-defensive and transparent with others and maintaining no secrecy (in Berne's imagery 'speaking Martian'). In an ideal situation where there is caring, trust and mutual respect, openness greatly facilitates social relations and the achievement of INTIMACY and is the attitude endorsed by transactional analysis.

In a few situations openness involves risks that must be balanced against potential gains; the aim is to remain open while keeping oneself safe. Openness or genuineness (in TA terminology, being in the OK:OK position, in Rogers' language being congruent or real) involves authenticity, self-awareness and awareness of the other and of the process in which both are involved from a non-judgemental and accepting position. This awareness needs to be shared but openness is compatible with maintaining some boundaries.

operationalise to put into action. In transactional analysis there are usually close links between theoretical concepts and therapeutic behaviours. This derives from the clarity of its theory and its incorporation of a behavioural perspective. It is therefore a system that can readily be operationalised.

options alternatives that may be chosen. When clients become stuck they may be unaware of options or they may be DISCOUNTING options. See DISCOUNT MATRIX.

options (Karpman's) Karpman (1971) suggested that there are wide choices available in the way we TRANSACT with others. If we wish to challenge the way the other person is behaving classical theory tells us that we can cross his or her TRANSACTION by replying from an ego-state other than the one that was addressed. Karpman highlighted the rich possibilities that arise if we make use of all the available FUNCTIONAL EGO-STATES. Very different options result, for example, from responding from the rebellious adapted Child, the Adult or the controlling Parent where a response from compliant adapted Child is expected. If we choose an ego-state, we make that choice in the Adult so there will be an element of 'as if' in our transacting, although the Adult will be able to shift cathexis into the chosen ego-state.

82

oral stage (psychoanalysis) in classical Freudian developmental theory the stage when the mouth is the main source of pleasurable experience and so is the primary erotogenic zone. In OBJECT RELATIONS theory it refers to the same period (first to second year of life) but the emphasis is on the baby's relationship first to the part-object of the breast and then to the object of the mother. In transactional analysis, the development of the schizoid PERSONALITY ADAPTATION is related to unresolved issues at the oral stage. In much of his writing Berne seemed to think of script formation as usually becoming fixed in the seven-year-old (post oedipal) child (although he was clearly aware of the importance of very early influences). Recent developments in transactional analysis, however, have shifted emphasis to earlier developmental stages such as the oral stage (a position that is more Kleinian/object relations than Freudian). See OBJECT.

organic illness illness in which there is malfunctioning of the body, as opposed to psychological illness (functional disorders) in which no such malfunction can be observed. Illnesses that manifest psychologically sometimes have physical causes (for example, anxiety states because of thyrotoxicosis). Some psychiatrists who adopt the MEDICAL MODEL suggest that physical causes will ultimately be found for most mental illnesses, however there is little evidence to support this view at present. Transactional analysts takes the view that most psychological problems have psychological causes while acknowledging the need to address physical (organic) issues. However, they also note the close connection between mind and body and that this connection can operate in both directions (i.e. psychological states can influence body functioning).

organisational transactional analysis transactional analysis applied to the study of organisations. See SPECIAL FIELDS.

outcome the end result of a process of change. The psychological situation of the client at the end of the process of counselling or psychotherapy. In transactional analysis a CONTRACT is made to seek a specific outcome, which is made as clear as possible, and in the final stage of therapy the achieved outcome is assessed by the client against the agreed objectives. The contractual process is not rigid and the contracted outcome can be (and often is) revised as the therapy proceeds.

outcome fantasies a useful technique when developing an outcome contract is to invite the client to fantasise the desired outcome in as much detail as possible ('What do you see? Who is there? How do you feel?' etc.). This also shifts thinking away from the negative (I want to be rid of my problem) to the positive (this is the way I want to be).

overadaptation a PASSIVE BEHAVIOUR in which great effort is put into adapting to the imagined needs and wishes of the other person. It involves the DISCOUNTING of one's own needs and of the ability of the other person to ask for what he or she wants.

overdetailing the use of excessive amounts of detail when, for example, answering a simple question. In the Schiffs' terminology this is a THINKING DISORDER and is a clue that DISCOUNTING is occurring. Energy is being shifted away from the here-and-now issues of communicating with the other person.

over-reactor an alternative name (in full 'enthusiastic over-reactor') for the histrionic (hysteric) PERSONALITY ADAPTATION.

83

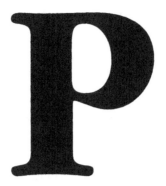

P₁ the Parent in the Child ego-state. This is an early ego-state that is formed in response to the rules given to the child by a parent figure. The child is not yet able to evaluate these rules but incorporates his or her understanding (or misunderstanding) of them rigidly. The child does not understand the consequences of disobeying the rules but fears that it may be very frightening (their world may become unsafe). As a result, a harsh, frightening figure is often created in P₁ by the child to frighten himself or herself into conformity. A number of negative names for P₁ reflect the harsh, negative content often found in P₁: Witch Parent, Ogre, Pig Parent. Grandiose positive versions of P₁ are also contacted, which are referred to as the Fairy Godmother, Good Fairy or Santa Claus. These also reflect the MAGICAL THINKING through which the child seeks to gain control over his or her world. The term Magical Parent includes both positive and negative aspects of P₁. Berne's term, 'the Electrode', refers to the way the Child responds almost compulsively to the rewards and punishments of P₁.

Melanie Klein describes a similar phenomenon but offers a somewhat different explanation. See SPLITTING.

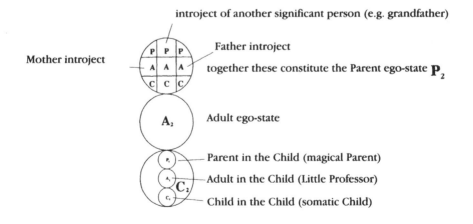

Figure 20 Second-order structural analysis (Berne, 1961).

P₂ the Parent ego-state proper. This contains behaviours, thought and feeling patterns of parent figures experienced in the past in the form of INTROJECTS of these individuals.

P₃ sometimes used for one of the Parent ego-states within the Parent ego-state (i.e. the Parent of an introject). The content is introjected material from a grandparent.

palimpsest literally a parchment on which old writing has been erased to make way for new. Sometimes the earlier writing would show through later. In transactional analysis the palimpsest is a later version of the script. This is developed in later childhood as the child draws on new potentialities.

parallel process it is often observed that when a counsellor or psychotherapist has SUPERVISION, the PROCESS of the supervision shows remarkable similarities to the process of the therapy that is being brought to supervision. For example, if the client has succeeded in setting up a game of DO ME SOMETHING with the therapist then the therapist may try to set up a similar game with the supervisor ('I really do not know what to do with this client, you must help me'). The supervision process parallels the therapy process. The issue brought by the supervisee to supervision will usually be one in which he or she feels stuck. This 'stuckness' results from the internalisation by the therapist or counsellor of the client's issues, for example by PROJECTIVE IDENTIFICATION by the client, or the issue may be one that the supervisee has not resolved and he or she is therefore caught in proactive COUNTER-TRANSFERENCE (Clarkson, 1992) with the client. The supervisee then takes these issues through into the supervision as if they were his or her own. This is a complex process and other factors may be involved. Identification of the paral-lel process is a powerful resource in effective supervision.

paranoid personality adaptation a personality pattern occurring in individuals who are able to function reasonably well, but who show some features of paranoid personality disorder. There is excessive suspiciousness of others and often a tendency to become isolated. It is characterised by a Be Perfect DRIVER. It can take two forms (Zeichnich, 1968). With the Child form of the driver 'I have to be perfect for you' others are seen as threatening and critical and withdrawn from (Victim position on the DRAMA TRIANGLE). With the Parent form of the driver 'You have to be perfect for me' the individual seeks to dominate and control others and may be extremely demanding and critical (Persecutor position on the Drama Triangle). People with this adaptation often seek positions of authority. See also PERSONALITY ADAPTATION, WARE SEQUENCE.

paranoid-schizoid position (Kleinian psychoanalysis) according to Melanie Klein, the small baby feels very vulnerable and exposed to potential annihilation. He or she is unable to cope with the negative aspects of the parent (when the parent has failed to meet the child's needs) as part of the total reality of that parent so splits off the negative from the positive. Melanie Klein referred to these as the good breast and the bad breast as she believed that at this stage the baby relates to the mother more as a breast (part object) than as a total person. The baby projects her anger with the bad breast on to the breast so that it seems to be attacking her. She responds to this from a withdrawn (schizoid) or angry attacking (paranoid) position. Ultimately the child realises that both aspects are part of the same person. As now love and hate are directed to the same person, love can mitigate hate (the mother is loved even when the child experiences her behaviour as frustrating). The child has achieved OBJECT CONSTANCY (understanding that the mother is one OBJECT and not two) and entered the DEPRESSIVE POSITION. The child now understands that his or her hate has been directed to the loved mother and feels remorse and the desire to make reparation. The resolution of the paranoid-schizoid position may not be completed in infancy so that it may contribute to later pathology. McDevitt and Mahler (1980) place this resolution as usually occurring at age three (associated with the individuation-separation crisis) although other Kleinians believe it can occur much earlier. Klein influenced Berne's thinking about life positions and offers an explanation of the observation that clients in therapy do not move directly from either the I+U− (paranoid) or I−U− (schizoid) life positions to the healthy position I+U+ without visiting the I−U+ (depressive) life position. See LIFE POSITIONS, OK CORRAL.

Parent ego-state usually written 'Parent'. The ego-state that contains behaviours, thoughts and feeling patterns of parent figures experienced in the past in the form of INTROJECTS of these individuals. In the PAC diagram it is shown by a circle containing the letter P. In second-order analysis of ego-states this main Parent ego-state is designated P_2.

Parent interview a therapeutic technique developed by McNeel (1976). The client is invited to project a Parent figure (introject) on to a chair. The client then sits on the chair and 'becomes' the introject, which is interviewed by the therapist. What happens is that, in effect, the therapist gives therapy to the introject. This has proved to be a very powerful technique that, in skilled hands, can facilitate profound changes. See also REPARENTING THE PARENT.

Parent resolution a therapeutic technique developed by Dashiel (1978) in which, after making an Adult:Adult contract with the client the therapist uses Gestalt technique (see CUSHION WORK) to separate ego-states. The Parent is then opened up and given new information, PERMISSIONS and opportunities or resolutions.

passive-aggressive personality adaptation a personality pattern characterised by rebelliousness coupled with a reluctance to initiate. The rebelliousness is usually expressed covertly by stubborn, resentful or manipulative behaviour. People with this pattern have not found it safe to ask openly and directly for their needs and wants as children. See PERSONALITY ADAPTATIONS, WARE SEQUENCE.

passive behaviours four behaviours identified by the Cathexis School (Schiff et al., 1975) as often resorted to under stress but not leading to problem resolution because of the DISCOUNTING of important aspects of reality. See FOUR PASSIVE BEHAVIOURS.

passivity unassertiveness, responding to a challenge by behaviours that do not give rise to problem solving because of DISCOUNTING of important aspects of reality. For example, in doing nothing the individual's power to effect change is being discounted probably together with other aspects of the situation (such as availability of options or resources). See FOUR PASSIVE BEHAVIOURS and DISCOUNT MATRIX.

pastimes a form of TIME STRUCTURING in which there is talk about a topic but no action is taken concerning it. Pastimes are not rigid, like RITUALS, but give considerable freedom without having to undertake the commitment to action involved in an ACTIVITY or the emotional involvement of GAMES. They constitute a large part of social activity and besides filling time they provide a milieu in which people can safely check each other out before becoming more involved.

patient the term used by doctors, psychiatrists and psychoanalysts for the people to whom they provide their services (derived from the Latin *patientia* – 'to bear', and so implying someone who suffers). We find it in the writings of Eric Berne who trained as a psychiatrist. Modern transactional analysts prefer the term 'client', signalling that the people who use their services make a free choice to do so.

payoff Berne (1972) wrote '[the script is] a life plan made in childhood, reinforced by the parents, justified by subsequent events, and culminating in a chosen alternative'. This suggests that one of the factors behind script behaviour is the unaware seeking of a negative outcome (the payoff) which has been decided in childhood. This offers a teleological view of script (that it is moving towards an end rather than being driven). Likewise games are seen as moving towards a payoff, the final outcome of the series of ULTERIOR TRANSACTIONS. To function, these payoffs must have something to offer, which may be a 'solution' in terms of Child logic of some life issue or some form of SECONDARY GAIN.

peer supervision the supervision of each other by psychotherapists of approximately equal skill and experience, as opposed to using a trained and experienced professional supervisor. This avoids creating a hierarchy and reduces expense but is likely to be less challenging and informative. Peer supervision cannot be counted towards the supervision requirement in training as a Certified Transactional Analyst.

performance anxiety anxiety that is linked to performing in public (for example, as a musician, sports-person etc.). More generally, anxiety felt whenever there is some demand from others for an outcome that the client fears she or he may not be able to provide. Factors that are often involved are the presence of Be Perfect and Please Others DRIVER MESSAGES and childhood experiences of SHAMING.

performing Tuckman's (1965) final stage of small-group development. Members give up some of their own proclivities in favour of group cohesion. The group is then able to concentrate its energy on its tasks. Clarkson (1992) has integrated Tuckman's theories with those of Berne (1963, 1966) and identifies the performing stage with Berne's *operative group imago*. See GROUPS, STAGES OF DEVELOPMENT.

Perls, Fritz with his wife Laura, the originator of GESTALT THERAPY. Gestalt has had a major influence on transactional analysis, particularly through the Gouldings' (1979) redecision therapy and Erskine and Moursund's (1988) integrative psychotherapy. Perls trained originally as a psychoanalyst but reacted against the analytic approach, which he saw as reductionist and over-intellectual, and sought in Gestalt therapy to develop an existential psychotherapy firmly based in the experience of the client and not on imposing theoretical abstractions on that experience.

permission a message that something is allowable and OK. It may be given verbally or behaviourally. A mother who holds her baby and smiles at her is giving permissions to exist and be close. A permission is the opposite of an INJUNCTION, which is a negative script message. The giving of permissions to neutralise the effects of script messages is an important aspect of psychotherapy and counselling. See also THREE Ps.

Persecutor (written with a capital) one of the three positions or roles on the DRAMA TRIANGLE (also known as the Karpman Triangle). The use of the capital distinguishes it from the ordinary use of the word. As with the other two positions, Victim and Rescuer, the Persecutor position involves DISCOUNTING. The Persecutor sees others as not-OK and therefore meriting his attacks.

person-centred counselling (or therapy) the name now preferred for Rogerian counselling or therapy (formerly often referred to as client-centred counselling). This approach to therapy and counselling was developed by Carl Rogers (1951, 1961). It is a humanistic approach whose core idea is that, if the conditions for change are created by the therapist then the client will change. The essential conditions for change are the CORE CONDITIONS of empathy, congruence and unconditional positive regard. According to Rogers, if these are created successfully then the client will become more aware, more flexible and fluid in their feelings, thoughts and actions, and less rigid and fixed. The client will develop an *internal locus of evaluation*, become more self-determining and less influenced by the perceived need to please others, to mask themselves and to live according to others' expectations. A trust in the client's ability to find his or her own solutions is essential in this approach. It sees interventionist therapies such as transactional analysis as likely to create an unequal relationship in which the client may be inhibited from seeking his or her own solutions and finding his or her own direction. It shares with transactional analysis the humanistic and existential perspectives and differs mainly in its idea that the therapist follows the client's lead rather than being more active in negotiating the direction of therapy.

personal development group a group in which personal issues can be explored safely in a supportive setting to achieve personal growth. This term is sometimes preferred to therapy group as the latter term implies that some form of treatment is received – i.e. that the group members have 'problems' that need to be 'treated'. Group work has always been important in transactional analysis (Berne, 1966) and was originally the dominant mode of working, but as the discipline has developed individual work has become increasingly important and is now the major therapeutic approach.

personal growth a HUMANISTIC THERAPY concept implying the realisation of the individual's potential for psychological, emotional and spiritual development. This avoids the medical concepts of malfunction, treatment and cure that still cling to psychotherapy and to some extent also to counselling. The 'inner drive to wholeness' is conceptualised in transactional analysis through the idea of PHYSIS.

personalisation believing that events or remarks relate to oneself. This is common in early childhood, especially during the age of MAGICAL THINKING. This remains a feature of the Child ego-state so some level of personalisation is common in normal subjects. In its extreme form it constitutes delusions of reference.

personality adaptation a term adopted by Ware (1983) to describe a structuring of the personality that is compatible with normal functioning but shows similarities to certain types of psychological disorder. He named the adaptations using psychiatric terminology (see DSM-IV). Each is the result of a specific pattern of early experiences reacted to by a characteristic pattern of defences. Personality adaptation theory is unusual in transactional analysis in being a SYNDROME approach (i.e. the concepts are based on a number of features that commonly occur together). Characteristically, in transactional analysis, diagnosis consists of identifying individual features of pathology (for example injunctions, counterinjunctions, games, rackets, etc.) rather than characteristic packages of such features. Ware's work has been extensively developed by Taibi Kahler, who based his process therapy approach on it, and by Vann Joines (1986, 1988). For a review of Kahler's approach see Stewart (1996b). Joines has proposed an alternative set of names for the adaptations to stress the fact that they represent 'normal' states and that there are positive aspects to each of the adaptations. The Ware (psychiatric) and Joines names for the adaptations are:

Obsessive-compulsive (workaholic)
Schizoid (creative dreamer)
Passive-aggressive (rebel)
Histrionic or hysteric (enthusiastic over-reactor)
Paranoid (brilliant sceptic)
Antisocial (charming manipulator)

Ware noted that clients responded differently to thinking, feeling and behavioural interventions. The order in which these are used is very significant. It is important to start with the function which is least defended (which he called the *open door*) and deal last with the function that is most defended (the *trap door,* so called because if it is addressed prematurely the consequent defensive reaction is often highly counter-therapeutic). The main thrust of the therapy needs to be towards the *target door*, that function which is only moderately defended. The sequence of therapy therefore follows the general pattern: open door, target door, trap door. The sequences he identified (Ware sequences) are:

- obsessive-compulsive (workaholic) driver Be Perfect, Ware sequence: thinking feeling, behaviour;

- schizoid (creative dreamer) driver Be Strong, Ware sequence: behaviour (passive), thinking, feeling;

- passive-aggressive (rebel) driver Try Hard, Ware sequence: behaviour (resistant), feeling, thinking;

- histrionic or hysteric (enthusiastic over-reactor) driver Please, Ware sequence: feeling, thinking, behaviour;

- paranoid (brilliant sceptic) driver Be Perfect (usually the Parent version 'you must be perfect for me'), Ware sequence: thinking, feeling, behaviour;

- antisocial (charming manipulator) driver Try Hard, Ware sequence: behaviour (manipulation), feeling, thinking. The Parent ego-state is weak, crazy or excluded.

More than one adaptation may be present simultaneously, particularly those adaptations that are developmentally early (*primary adaptations* – schizoid and paranoid), commonly found with one of the later *secondary adaptations*.

Ware sequences should not be applied rigidly. They specify the probability of a 'door' being open at a particular stage of therapy (for example, an open door at the beginning, a trap door only at the end) but it is important for the therapist to monitor and respond to the client's current state. Under stress clients revert to their 'trap door' defences so the obsessive-compulsive client, for example, will often alternate between thinking (their usual 'open door' defence) and rigid behaviour (their ultimate 'trap door' defence). For further details see individual entries.

personality disorder (also character disorder). A psychological disorder in which the client lacks insight and tends to attribute his or her problems to others and to external circumstances and adopts maladaptive patterns of relating to his or her social environment. More generally, a class of behavioural disorders other than psychoses (in which there is disconnection from reality generally and not just social reality) and neuroses (in which there is insight into the ownership of the problem) in which the whole personality is involved and there is often relatively little anxiety or distress.

personality theory any theory that claims to explain individual characteristics, differences and different patterns of reacting to the environment. There are many such theories within the diverse schools of psychology. Transactional analysis, through its use of the ego-state model, is a theory of personality as well as a theory of interpersonal interaction.

phallic stage (psychoanalysis) the stage in Freud's theory of psychosexual development in which the child shows great interest in his penis or her clitoris. This follows the ANAL STAGE and precedes the OEDIPAL STAGE (i.e. at about three). Freud's stage terminology is sometimes used by transactional analysts e.g. Levin (1974).

phantasy (Kleinian psychoanalysis) unconscious images generated from the infant's own feelings and perceptions and not necessarily having any correlate in the external world (in contrast to *fantasy*, which consists of representations of the real world).

phenomenology the phenomenological approach consists in looking at the world 'from the inside' (what it 'feels' like to the individual) rather than what it looks like to an observer (the characteristic position of the scientific approach). Phenomenology derives from the work of the German philosopher Edmund Husserl (1859–1938) who advocated the study of immediate experience as the basis of psychology. The emphasis is on how events are perceived and experienced rather than on the events in the external world that generate these perceptions and experiences. Transactional analysis is a 'two-person psychology'. To achieve this it has to combine an external objective view (as in observing transactions) with an insight into the internal (phenomenological) perspective of the individual. This synthesis is achieved via ego-state theory. In diagnosing ego-states Berne specified four criteria, one of which is phenomenological. See EGO-STATE DIAGNOSIS.

phenomenological diagnosis of ego-states diagnosis on the basis of the client's report of his or her internal states (what he or she is thinking and feeling) and their resemblance to previous internal states (is this how it felt when you were five?).

philosophy of transactional analysis central to the philosophy of transactional analysis is the concept of the healthy life position: 'I'm OK, You're OK'. This means that I have accepted myself as I am as intrinsically valuable and I accept you similarly as you are. This does not mean that I consider every aspect of you or myself as entirely satisfactory, it is an evaluation of the whole self. This corresponds closely to Rogers' concept of unconditional positive regard. The second key concept is autonomy, being in charge of one's own life, interacting respectfully, caringly and contactfully with others but making one's own choices without being restrained by other people, whether present in the here-and-now or through internalised INTROJECTS.

Everyone is able to think for himself or herself and should be allowed to do so. Children should be encouraged to think and decide for themselves as far as they are able. Autonomy requires clear and open communication, which transactional analysis seeks to promote through its analysis of communication patterns. Eric Berne wrote about speaking and understanding Martian. Martians represent people who have not been initiated into the social patterns of our civilisation so that they see interactions as they really are. They say exactly what they mean as they see no reason to do otherwise. To listen for the Martian is to read the true message under its social presentation. The transactional analysis autonomy concept has much in common with Rogers' congruence. Associated with autonomy is the concept of PHYSIS, an inner drive to wholeness that moves the person to his or her own personal fulfilment, which cannot be chosen for them by anyone else. Rogers' third core condition, empathy, is not specifically addressed in the early literature of transactional analysis although it is implicit in it. It has always been a feature of the way most transactional analysts work, and follows from the humanistic viewpoint that underlies the discipline. It is perhaps this gap in the literature that made it possible for an intrusive, over-confrontational and non-empathic style of doing transactional analysis to flourish for a time among a few therapists in the 1970s. For recent work on empathy see Clark (1991). See also CORE CONDITIONS, CONFRONTATION.

phobia an irrational fear of some object, creature or situation, such as a fear of spiders (which in the UK are harmless) or open spaces. A phobia arises from Child CONTAMINATION of Adult. The fear in the Child ego-state is then experienced as if it related to current reality.

physis a drive towards wholeness and health that Berne (1957, 1972) symbolised by a vertical arrow passing through all three ego-states. This closely corresponds to the self-actualising principle of humanistic theory, implying both the possibility of personal growth and a natural tendency to pursue it. The concept derives from the ancient Greek philosopher Heraclitus and originally meant change or growth that comes from the spirit within the person (Liddell and Scott, 1935). For a discussion of this concept see Clarkson (1992).

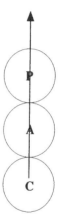

Figure 21 Physis illustrated as the aspiration arrow.

Piaget, Jean Swiss psychologist noted for his work on the cognitive development of children. See OBJECT PERMANENCE.

Pig Parent a derogatory term for the negative aspect of the Magical Parent, the Parent in the Child ego-state. See P_1

placement a period of practical, supervised work undertaken by a psychotherapy or counselling trainee in an agency other than his or her training base. Transactional analysis psychotherapy trainees are required to serve a placement in a psychiatric hospital or comparable institution before they can proceed to the Certified Transactional Analysis examination.

This enables them to become familiar with severe forms of psychological disturbance and to learn how to work alongside other mental health professionals.

plastic strokes positive gestures towards others (acts of recognition) that are clearly insincere, for example flattery. See STROKE.

Please the PLEASE DRIVER is often referred to as Please.

Please driver a behavioural pattern that seeks approval from others. This may show through a variety of behaviours, e.g. smiling (usually tensely), checking with others 'all right by you?', high-pitched voice rising at the end of the sentence, etc. The driver is a behavioural manifestation of a DRIVER MESSAGE, which is a component of script, so when driver behaviour is being shown the individual is in script. See PLEASE ME and PLEASE OTHERS.

Please me the Parent form of the PLEASE DRIVER. Drivers are most often encountered in their Child form, that is the individual replays a Parent message to himself or herself and responds from Child by seeking to conform to the message. However, the person may identify with the Parent ego-state and give the message to someone else. The Child form of the driver is (I Must) Please (You). The Parent form is (You Must) Please (Me).

Please others a way of specifying the Child form of the PLEASE DRIVER.

Poor Me a game initiated from the Victim position in which others are invited to be sympathetic so that they can be manipulated.

positive stroke a positive act of recognition such as a smile, a touch, a phrase – 'I like you'. See STROKE.

post-traumatic stress disorder (PTSD) a psychological disorder that follows exposure to unavoidable major damaging or life-threatening events. It may occur immediately after the events or its onset may be delayed, sometimes for long periods. It is characterised by repeated intrusive memories of the event (flashbacks and nightmares). Flashbacks and anxiety (which may reach the level of panic attacks) may be triggered by similar circumstances to those that accompanied or preceded the traumatic events, so there is commonly avoidance of such situations. There may be persistent anxiety and sleep disturbances. Defences against this may produce flattening of affect (numbing).

Psychotherapeutic interventions include re-experiencing the event in fantasy in a supportive environment. Because of the profound effects of an unsupported experience of trauma it may have a wide range of psychological consequences calling for a broad approach in which many of the therapeutic techniques of transactional analysis may need to be deployed. Therapy may also involve addressing earlier unresolved issues that have been reactivated by the traumatic event. The stress generated by the trauma can lead to regression so that the traumatisation may be recorded in a Child ego-state and at an earlier developmental stage than that at which it occurred. Much work with abuse survivors is in effect working with post-traumatic stress disorder.

potency the power of the therapist, as perceived by the client, to give permissions to overrule negative messages from the client's Parent ego-state. See THREE PS.

potential that which is capable of being but is not yet realised. Humanistic counselling lays great emphasis on human potential. Transactional analysis is rooted in humanistic values. In Eric Berne's symbolism, even if we are frogs we are capable of becoming princes and princesses. It is the function of the transactional analysis therapist to facilitate this change. The transactional analysis concept of PHYSIS refers to a drive to fulfil potential.

power the achievement of personal power (the ability to effect change) is essential if the client is to achieve AUTONOMY, which is a major aim of TA therapy. Counsellors and psychotherapists seek to empower their clients. Power in this sense is centred in the person, unlike political power, which is centred in groups and organisations and may seek to restrict autonomy.

preconscious (psychoanalysis) the part of the mind that contains material which can readily become conscious although it is not currently so (as opposed to the UNCONSCIOUS, whose content is very difficult to contact). This term is preferred by Freudians to SUBCONSCIOUS although the meaning is essentially the same. In transactional analysis these terms are usually avoided and 'out of awareness' used instead. This does not go beyond what can be observed and does not imply the existence of specific zones (preconscious, unconscious) in the mind.

prejudice a judgement or opinion formed beforehand without consideration of the facts. Prejudice is due to Parent CONTAMINATION of the Adult ego-state. A belief in the Parent ego-state deriving from an authority figure (usually in childhood) is misperceived as valid in current reality. See CONTAMINATION.

pressure of speech excessively fast speech in which the words seem to tumble over each other. This probably indicates a HURRY UP DRIVER. If severe it may be a sign of HYPOMANIA and therefore indicate MANIC-DEPRESSIVE disorder;

however, rapid speech may have been learned socially and may not be an indicator of a psychological problem.

primal wound there are four major types of psychological damage that are likely to result from inappropriate or abusive parenting. Adrienne Lee (1988b) calls these the four primal wounds, basing the concept on an idea of Mary Goulding. In all cases of serious psychological disturbance one or more primal wounds will be identifiable in the history. The four primal wounds are:

- *Abandonment* where the child has been left unsupported because of the physical absence of the parent.
- *Non-involvement* where the parent was physically present but did not make contact with the child, leaving him or her emotionally abandoned.
- *Engulfment* where the parent was intrusive and did not give the child space to be himself or herself and to individuate. This may take many forms, some clearly abusive (such as physical abuse or domineering behaviour) while others at first sight may appear benign (such as over-nurturance). See SECOND-ORDER SYMBIOSIS.
- *Hurt* which is actively abusive behaviour (physical, emotional or sexual abuse). Often what is happening is that the parent deals with his or her own emotional conflicts by PROJECTING on to the child (blaming). PROJECTIVE IDENTIFICATION (projecting *into* so that the other owns the projection) may also be occurring. Other primal wounds are likely to be found with hurt (for example, engulfment and non-involvement).

Early identification of primal wound helps the therapist or counsellor to match his or her style to the client's needs and avoid re-enacting the client's major issues in the therapy.

For example, a cool and detached style may re-enact non-involvement while a very involving style may be perceived as threatening by a client with engulfment issues. See also MODELS.

primary process thinking (psychoanalysis) Freud's concept of unconscious mental activity associated with the ID. It is characterised by the pleasure principle (a pursuit of pleasure and avoidance of pain without regard for the limitations of reality), a disregard for space and time and a tendency to combine thoughts and images (condensation) and to displace feelings from one person to another. These features are observable in the content of dreams. This concept is useful in understanding the sometimes bizarre nature of Child ego-state thinking. See SECONDARY PROCESS.

Principles of Group Treatment one of the major texts of transactional analysis. This book by Eric Berne, first published in 1966, is a major source of information on Berne's ideas about professional practice using transactional analysis, particularly as applied to group therapy. It also contains some development of the thinking about group processes, which he began in THE STRUCTURE AND DYNAMICS OF ORGANISATIONS AND GROUPS (1963).

process what happens in counselling or psychotherapy, as opposed to what is discussed, which is the CONTENT. Usually the process is the more psychologically significant. This is the meaning of Berne's THIRD RULE OF COMMUNICATION.

process model an integrative theory bringing together many aspects of transactional analysis. It was developed by Taibi Kahler and makes use of Paul Ware's concept of PERSONALITY ADAPTATIONS. For a summary of his approach see Stewart (1996b).

process script the characteristic process through which the script is expressed in action. This is shaped by the DRIVER MESSAGES. These are essentially messages about how to please the parents in childhood which are used to generate phoney (spurious) OKness in adult life to counteract the negative effect of INJUNCTIONS. Because the driver messages (counterinjunctions) specify behaviours that are supposed to elicit the approval of others (and more importantly of the internal Parent) it is these that shape the outward form of the script although the significant content of the script, which is responsible for most of the damage it causes, lies in the injunctions. As a result, people with very different pathology may express their scripts in similar ways (employ similar defences). However, the underlying pathology of the injunctions will affect the DEGREE of the script (the level of damage to self and others that occurs).

Each script process type can be characterised by a Greek myth and a slogan (Berne, 1970, 1972; Kahler, 1978). For example, the process script type which has the Be Perfect driver message is an Until script. People with this type of scripting respond to the internal message 'you can't get your needs met until you have done everything *perfectly*'. For example, they will not sit down to watch the TV until they have washed and dried the dishes and tidied the kitchen. The corresponding Greek myth is of Hercules, who had to perform a long series of incredibly difficult tasks before he was allowed to become immortal. The seven process scripts are listed below with their slogans and characteristic driver patterns.

- always (why does this always happen to me?). Try Hard.
- until (I can't do X until I have finished Y). Be Perfect.
- never (I never get what I most want). Be Strong.
- after (after the good times will come the bad). Please.

- almost I (I never quite make it). Please and Try Hard.
- almost II (I make it but move the goal posts so stay dissatisfied). Please and Be Perfect.
- open-ended (I run out of script and do not know what to do when a role ends). Please and Be Perfect.

procrastination putting things off. A failure to engage with an issue that is a source of internal conflict. There may be inactivity or effort may be directed into irrelevant behaviour that is unrelated to problem solving. This is frequently a sign of the PASSIVE-AGGRESSIVE PERSONALITY ADAPTATION that is characterised by the TRY HARD DRIVER.

program a 'how to' message from the contaminated Adult of a parent to the contaminated Adult of a child. This will provide information in support of scripty behaviour e.g. 'this is how to drink heavily' or 'this is how to alienate people'. Note that the Adult is contaminated, although this is not shown in the SCRIPT MATRIX diagram. Uncontaminated Adult is not involved in script. See also MESSAGE FORMAT.

progress Eric Berne (1966) warned against the 'making progress' approach in therapy using the metaphor that this consists in making frogs more comfortable rather than getting on with turning them back into princesses and princes. See FROGS INTO PRINCES.

projection a defence mechanism in which some aspect of the self that is unacceptable to the person is attributed to someone else. This often manifests as the blaming and criticising of others. It is the main defence of the PARANOID PERSONALITY ADAPTATION.

projective identification (Kleinian psychoanalysis) expelling part of the internal world (self or OBJECTS) into another person (external object) so that they identify with the projected feeling or thought as if it was their own. This constitutes projection *into* the other while simple projection is projection *on to* the other. This is particularly important with babies where verbal communication is absent. If the mother is able to take in the baby's feelings she can be intuitively aware of its needs and so be attuned (see ATTUNEMENT). Where the projection is negative the good mother can take this in and give out a positive response so that the baby's experience is positively transformed. Although this is not a transactional analysis concept, it has attracted interest among transactional analysts. The concept of projective identification also provides an alternative explanation of GAMES. Projective identification may also occur in therapy complicating the TRANSFERENCE and COUNTERTRANSFERENCE. A process similar to a parent's positive use of projective identification may occur in therapy. In this case the therapist will function in Bollas' (1987) terminology as a TRANSFORMATIONAL OBJECT. The transfer of script by projective identification between parent and child is probably the mechanism behind the EPISCRIPT.

protection therapeutic procedures to protect the client from the adverse effects of negative script elements during therapy. Therapy involves dismantling the defensive structure that underlies the script. This may leave the client vulnerable to injunctions or other toxic P_1 or P_2 material. An important aspect of protection is the closure of ESCAPE HATCHES. See THREE PS.

protocol the earliest version of the script incorporating the earliest memories and decisions. c.f. PALIMPSEST.

Provisional Teaching and Supervising Transactional Analyst see PTSTA.

psyche the mental apparatus.

psychiatry the medical speciality which deals with mental disorders. Psychiatrists may use a variety of therapeutic techniques including psychotherapy but often stress the medical aspects of mental disorder and the importance of medical interventions such as the use of psychotropic drugs and, in certain conditions, physical interventions such as ECT. c.f. PSYCHOTHERAPY, PSYCHOLOGY.

psychic energy in the PSYCHODYNAMIC model of mental processes these are understood in terms of flows of psychic energy (CATHEXIS) between structures in the PSYCHE. This concept is also employed in transactional analysis which has roots in the psychodynamic theories of Freud. Psychic energy is a metaphor used in describing intrapsychic processes and must be distinguished from physical energy. See ENERGY.

psychic organ a structure within the PSYCHE with a specific function. Freud postulated three psychic organs, the EGO, SUPEREGO and ID. In his original exposition of transactional analysis (1961) Berne postulated three psychic organs, the EXTEROPSYCHE, NEOPSYCHE and ARCHEOPSYCHE. These had the functions of 'generating' (were manifested phenomenologically as) the three types of ego-state, Parent, Adult and Child. In later writings this concept tended to be subsumed within the ego-state concept and the psychic organ concept has been little used in transactional analysis. However, it is sometimes important to make the distinction between psychic organs and ego-states. Despite their similarity to Freud's psychic organs, there is no direct correspondence between the concepts. See Novey (1997).

psychoanalysis the theories and clinical techniques deriving from the work of Sigmund Freud. This is a PSYCHODYNAMIC approach. Freud developed his theory over a long lifetime and his work has been extensively developed, reinterpreted and extended, so psychoanalysis constitutes a rich and diverse field of theory and practice although psychoanalysts share many assumptions and approaches. There are four major schools of psychoanalysis (name in brackets is the person who had the major influence in establishing the approach).

Drive theory (Freud)
Object relations (Fairbairn developing the ideas of Melanie Klein)
Ego psychology (Hartmann)
Self psychology (Kohut)

Berne trained as a psychoanalyst and much psychoanalytic thinking has been incorporated into transactional analysis. Often the original abstract psychoanalytic term was dropped or little used and replaced by a name for an observable phenomenon. For example, in the early literature of transactional analysis there are few references to transference but numerous references to phenomena caused by transference (such as games, script, rubber-banding, 'putting a face on' etc.). The language had moved sharply towards the concrete. This made it refreshingly down-to-earth, objective and accessible. However, as transactional analysis developed, it found the lack of an abstract language an increasing liability and also became aware that it had isolated itself from important developments in theory such as self psychology. Probably the watershed was crossed with Moiso's (1985) article on ego-states and transference and there is now a growing interest in integrating psychoanalytic thinking into transactional analysis. The areas of psychoanalysis that have drawn the most interest are post-Freudian and particularly recent developments in object relations and self psychology. See PSYCHOANALYTIC RENAISSANCE.

psychoanalytic renaissance term used by Stewart (1996a) to describe the renewed interest in psychoanalytic theory that has characterised much recent thinking in transactional analysis.

psychodrama a method of PSYCHOTHERAPY in which the client joins with a group in expressing and working through their issues through improvised drama. The approach was developed by Moreno and influenced GESTALT THERAPY and through it transactional analysis which derives techniques (for example, CUSHION WORK used in REDECISION THERAPY) from psychodrama.

psychodynamic an approach that uses theoretical models of intrapsychic process that deal with the interplay of forces and the flow of PSYCHIC ENERGY (cathexis) between intrapsychic structures. PSYCHOANALYSIS (Freud) and analytical psychology (Jung) are the two major psychodynamic approaches. Eric Berne trained as a psychoanalyst and transactional analysis uses psychodynamic models (for example, the flow of energy or cathexis between ego-states) although these have been integrated with humanistic (for example, the 'I'm OK, You're OK' position, physis) and cognitive-behavioural approaches (for example, analysis of transactions). The main integrating idea has been the concept of the ego-state.

psychological level in an ULTERIOR TRANSACTION the implicit message that in fact determines the outcome of the transaction, c.f. SOCIAL LEVEL.

psychology the scientific study of the mind in all its aspects. Psychology is applied in many fields in addition to the clinical field; c.f. PSYCHIATRY, PSYCHOTHERAPY.

psychopathology a general term for any kind of psychological disturbance, major or minor.

psychosis a mental disorder in which contact is lost with external (consensual) reality and the client mistakes his or her internal world for the real world. Clients may suffer from DELUSIONS (false beliefs) about themselves and others as well as disturbances of sensory perception resulting in HALLUCINATION (for example, seeing or hearing things which are not 'there' in consensual reality). Once lost in their internal world, clients have no objective measures of scale so delusions are often grandiose. Psychosis may be a reaction to extreme stress (brief reactive psychosis), in which case it may be an isolated experience. Repeated attacks of psychosis indicate more serious psychological problems. A person in psychosis is putting insufficient CATHEXIS into Adult to maintain contact with reality. Delusions and hallucinations derive from Child and Parent material that the Adult is not processing. Traditional transactional analysis cannot be used to work with people in psychosis since it requires the co-operation of the Adult. Moreover, transactional analysis is a contractual process and without a functional Adult the psychotic client cannot enter into a valid contract. The Schiffs (CATHEXIS SCHOOL) developed methods for using transactional analysis with psychotic clients and claimed a high level of success. See REPARENTING.

psychosomatic certain physical illnesses are believed to be linked to psychological states. There is evidence that some cases of eczema, migraine, asthma and colitis are affected by psychological factors and a psychological component has been suggested in many other conditions. An illness that involves both mind and body is termed psychosomatic. The Child in the Child ego-state C_1 (see EGO-STATE, SECOND-ORDER

ANALYSIS) is referred to as the *somatic child*. At the stage when this early ego-state develops existence is more centred on the body than it is in later stages of childhood. Transactional analysis regards psychosomatic illness as indicative of damage at this level. If conditions involve mind and body then they can be treated via either route and perhaps best by both. Speculation on the psychosomatic origin of disease should not therefore preclude the use of physical methods of treatment. See BODY SCRIPTING.

psychotherapy treatment of psychological problems by talking to the client. There are many schools of psychotherapy but these fall into a relatively small number of types and despite the disagreement in which theorists sometimes engage, there is widespread agreement about general principles. In the UK there is a governing body to which most major psychotherapy training organisations belong: the United Kingdom Council for Psychotherapy. Trainees who satisfy the standards of any body that is a full member are placed on the National Register of Psychotherapists. The UK transactional analysis organisation, the Institute of Transactional Analysis, is a full member of the UKCP so certified transactional analysts with a clinical speciality become UKCP registered psychotherapists when they qualify.

Each discipline has a theory of the structure of mind and of the nature of mental processes, and most of these derive from, or have been strongly influenced by the work of, Sigmund Freud. The splitting into disciplines has not been unproductive – it has resulted in many people looking at the problems posed by the human condition in a great variety of ways. Integrative therapies have developed in which insights of diverse disciplines have been brought together. Transactional analysis is such an approach drawing on psychodynamic, humanistic and behaviourist sources. The term COUNSELLING overlaps with psychotherapy and counsellors and psychotherapists draw on similar theory and make use of similar techniques. The exact boundary between these two disciplines remains a subject of debate.

psychotropic drugs medical drugs that give rise to change of mood. These include antipsychotic drugs or major tranquillisers such as chlorpromazine, also anxiolytics such as the benzodiapines (commonly referred to as tranquillisers) which reduce anxiety and antidepressants, which affect mood only. Drugs are useful for handing crisis situations or the seriously disturbed client but they may interfere with psychotherapy by making Adult less available and by blocking feelings thus lowering the motivation to change and obstructing access to Child.

PTSD see POST-TRAUMATIC STRESS DISORDER.

PTSTA Provisional Teaching and Supervising Transactional Analyst. A certified transactional analyst who has been endorsed as able to give officially recognised transactional analysis training and supervision at a TEW (training endorsement workshop). A PTSTA is required to have regular supervision from a TSTA (teaching and supervising transactional analyst).

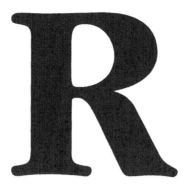

racket also **rackety** (adjective.) Unauthentic and manipulative. See RACKET BEHAVIOUR and RACKET FEELING.

racket (noun) (1) A racket behaviour. (2) A response that substitutes for a feeling. For example, a confusion racket is where a feeling of confusion substitutes for an authentic feeling such as anger. An anger racket is where anger substitutes for another feeling such as fear.

racket behaviour also **racketeering** a behaviour or sequence of behaviours that results in feeling a racket feeling. This is based on behaviours learned and encouraged in childhood, which were early strategies for having stroking and other needs met. Racket behaviour has a manipulative quality but the manipulation is out of awareness. Fanita English (1971) distinguishes four styles of racketeering: Helpless, Bratty (in Britain this is called 'Whingy'), Helpful and Bossy. Although they may have been successful in childhood, racket behaviours are a very unsatisfactory way of having needs met in the adult world. Rackets derive from and reinforce script. Rackets resemble GAMES, which also result in the participants feeling racket feelings. There are two major differences: a racket can be played one-handed, that is a situation can be set up that will result in the person feeling racket feelings without involving anyone else (e.g. by losing something), whereas games always involve two or more people. There is also no role-switch on the DRAMA TRIANGLE. Racketeering can proceed indefinitely whereas GAMES move inevitably to the SWITCH and CROSSUP. English has suggested that a game is a racket that has moved into an unstable state.

racket feelings unauthentic feelings involving the substitution of one feeling for another (English, 1971). This substitution is done out of awareness, (for example, crying when angry; getting angry when scared). A racket feeling has been learned and encouraged as a way of having stroking and other needs met in childhood and is accepted as a way of discharging emotion, whereas expression of the authentic feelings has been discouraged. The substituted feeling may be one of the four primary authentic feelings – sadness, anger, fear or happiness; one of the complex (and unhelpful) feelings that involve both thinking and feeling (are affective and cognitive) such as guilt and shame; or a non-affective state of mind such as confusion or blankness.

racket system a dynamic model of scripts as interlocking, self-reinforcing systems of racket behaviours and script beliefs, developed by Erskine and Zalcman (1979). It is now often referred to as the *script system*. Major elements in the system are Script Beliefs, Repressed Feelings, manifestations of script (racket behaviours), which the authors describe as Rackety Displays, and Reinforcing Memories. Rackety Displays are subdivided into Observable (observable to an external observer), Internal Experiences and Fantasies. Each part reinforces the other parts, setting up a dynamic system. This model differs markedly from Steiner's SCRIPT MATRIX. Steiner's model is static and answers the questions 'how did the script originate and what is its content?' whereas Erskine and Zalcman's model answers the question 'how is the script maintained and what is its process?' The models are complementary and each offers an invaluable basis for treatment planning, see Figure 22. For an up-dated view of the racket system and racket analysis see Zalcman (1990).

rackety (adjective) appertaining to a RACKET. Having the qualities of a RACKET or of RACKETEERING.

rage extreme anger. Melanie Klein believed that all babies at times per-ceived their caretakers as persecutory and felt rage towards them. Transactional analysts (and therapists of certain other modalities) sometimes use rage-reduction techniques that involve inviting the client to get in touch with repressed rage and grief occasioned by bonding failures and abusive relationships. This is done contractually (see CONTRACT) and in an environment that is both physically and emotionally safe. See CATHARSIS, ANGER WORK.

rapo a GAME in which a sexual advance is at first invited and then repulsed. The other party is switched from the position of Rescuer (providing what is asked for) to Victim while being invited into guilt by being accused of being a Persecutor. This is a sexual version of NIGYYSOB.

rapport an understanding relationship between client and therapist that enables the client to feel safe, connected and responded to. The early establishment of rapport is essential if an effective therapeutic relationship is to be established. See also EMPATHY, THERAPEUTIC ALLIANCE.

rapprochement crisis (psychoanalysis – object relations) Margaret Mahler's term for the developmental stage in which the child deals with establishing

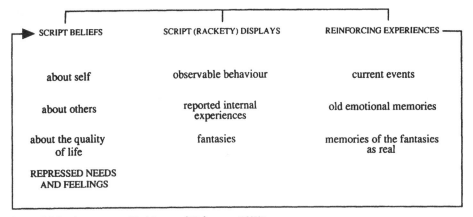

Figure 22 Racket system (Erskine and Zalcman, 1979).

his or her own separate identity from the mother while maintaining the relationship. According to OBJECT RELATIONS theory this calls for a new type of relationship (relationship to the mother as OBJECT), which brings together the child's opposing wishes for merger and autonomy. This is also associated with the achievement of libidinal OBJECT CONSTANCY (the frustrating and nurturant aspects of the mother are recognised as derived from one person so love is able to mitigate hate). This stage is often stormy and reaches its height at age two to three, so is often referred to as 'the terrible twos'. Levin (1974) identifies this stage with the emergence of the Adult ego-state. Problems at this stage are associated with the establishment of the PASSIVE-AGGRESSIVE and OBSESSIVE-COMPULSIVE PERSONALITY ADAPTATIONS (Joines, 1986).

rationalisation a process in which a reason is found for an action after it has been decided on, thus justifying it and concealing its true motivation.

reaction formation (psychoanalysis) a defence in which an unacceptable impulse is controlled by exaggerating its opposite. For example, impulses to behave in violent and cruel ways may be controlled by manifesting an exaggerated gentleness and solicitude.

real self that part of the personality experienced as 'me'. This may not be the same as the part that is in control of behaviour, which is known as the *executive*. According to Berne (1961) the real self is that part of the personality that has the most free energy, whereas in the executive the sum of free energy and unbound energy is the greatest. See ENERGY, CATHEXIS.

reality, consensual the Cathexis (Schiff et al., 1975) term for the view of reality

that we share with others on the basis of shared experience of the world.

reality, internal (personal) our personal experience of existence. This is no less real than consensual reality; in fact it feels more so. My pain, my fear are uniquely part of my experience, others may sympathise but they cannot feel them. In order to deal with others and the world effectively I must be able to distinguish between personal reality and CONSENSUAL REALITY. Failure to do so (if I believe others can feel my pain or think my thoughts or vice versa) results in PSYCHOSIS.

reality testing checking beliefs against our own perceptions and those of others (that the world is the way we think it is). This is one of the major functions of the Adult ego-state. PSYCHOSIS involves a major breakdown in reality testing so that the client's INTERNAL REALITY is confused with CONSENSUAL REALITY. See Schiff et al. (1975).

rebel this term is often preferred to describe the PASSIVE-AGGRESSIVE PERSONALITY ADAPTATION.

rebellious Child a functional manifestation of the Child ego-state. Usually regarded as an aspect of the adapted Child. The rebellious Child's responses are determined by the parents although in a negative way i.e. the child does the opposite of what he or she believes the parent wants him or her to do. The child has learned that the most effective way of obtaining STROKES from their parents is to oppose them. Often written 'Rebellious Child'. See FUNCTIONAL Ego-stateS.

rebirthing a therapeutic technique sometimes employed in transactional analysis (as well as other therapeutic modalities). It involves a symbolic repetition of the birth experience. Therapeutic aims include dealing with birth trauma, providing an opportunity to give permissions and affirmations that were absent in the original experience and also to provide the sense of a new beginning and therefore the potentiality to choose new paths through life, see Grof 1985.

rechilding a therapeutic technique for generating new Child ego-state to provide a resource for integrated Adult functioning (Clarkson and Fish, 1988). The client is invited to regress to an age at which he or she had experiential or developmental deficits and allows himself or herself to create new Child ego-states with positive responses to a wide variety of situations. This provides a corrective experience that is lodged in the newly created Child ego-state but that becomes a historical reality for the integrated Adult.

reciprocity a balanced interaction between two people in which there is mutuality and an equality of power, influence and openness to the other. Ideally a therapeutic relationship should involve reciprocity; however, the client often feels powerless when he or she enters therapy and has perceived the therapist as someone who has the power to help them. Transactional analysis stresses the importance of promoting AUTONOMY and empowering the client. The process of making a CONTRACT is important in this, as also is the sharing of theory with the client.

recognition hunger a need for recognition by others that is met at the most basic level in the infant by physical contact (Berne, 1961). Normal psychological development is impossible without some satisfaction of the hunger and the search for recognition is a major motivator. See STIMULUS HUNGER, STROKING, STRUCTURE HUNGER.

record keeping the making of clinical notes on clients. This is stressed in the training of therapists and is a part of good professional practice, enabling the therapist to maintain an overview of the therapy and keep track of important points and changes. Record keeping raises issues regarding CONFIDENTIALITY, particularly where the therapist is not working independently but within an organisation. It is important that these are dealt with in establishing the THERAPY CONTRACT. It may be necessary to have a three-cornered contract in which the contracts between the therapist and the organisation and the client and the organisation are also made clear. Berne (1966) recommends drawing up an organisational diagram charting all the external influences on the therapeutic relationship.

redecision changing a script decision. Therapeutic procedures for facilitating redecision are central to the REDECISION SCHOOL of transactional analysis.

redecision school one of the major schools of transactional analysis based on the work of Robert and Mary Goulding (1972, 1976). Script is a response to EARLY LIFE DECISIONS. As the individual strives for autonomy, these set up internal conflicts known as IMPASSES. There are three types of impasse (originally referred to as degrees of impasse). Type one concerns COUNTERINJUNCTIONS, these are messages about how to be OK given by parents (for example, Please – you are OK if you please your parents or others, or Be Perfect – you are OK if you get *everything* right). As the individual begins to become aware of how the decision to respond to these messages conflicts with his or her needs, the individual experiences an impasse. Type two impasses relate to INJUNCTIONS, messages given (usually out of awareness) by parents when they respond to their own unresolved Child needs at the expense of the child. The Gouldings identified 12 typical forms that these messages take such as Don't Exist, Don't Be You or Don't Be Important. Type three impasses relate to basic issues around identity. The Gouldings gave a theoretical account of the mechanism of the impasses in terms of second-order structural analysis of ego-states. There is disagreement among transactional analysts about how impasses are best represented and MELLOR (1980) has proposed an alternative theory that incorporates a developmental perspective and also avoids the switch from a structural to a functional model in the Gouldings' representation of the type 3 impasse. See IMPASSE.

The Gouldings developed a therapeutic technique for impasse resolution that incorporates GESTALT technique. A conflict issue is identified and the antagonist (usually an aspect of a parent or authority figure) is projected on to a chair or cushion. The client is facilitated in entering into a dialogue from Child but retaining the support of his or her own Adult. The client may take either position by moving between the chairs or cushions. If the resolution is successful a new decision is taken from Child resulting in a movement out of script.

redefining   a response that shifts the issue from the one being addressed, often by responding to a question by the answer to a different question; for example 'What do you *feel* when I say that?' 'I *think* I shall have to try harder to get it right.' This type of redefining transaction is called a TANGENTIAL TRANSACTION as it goes off in a new direction. There is another type called a BLOCKING TRANSACTION where the issue is avoided by disagreeing with its meaning or purpose, e.g. 'How do you feel when I say that?' 'I'm not sure what you mean by feeling, do you mean physically?' People use redefining transactions to maintain their view of themselves, others and the world – that is, to stay in script. Redefining involves DISCOUNTING and serves to maintain SYMBIOSIS, an

unhealthy dependence on others in which the resources of the personality are not fully used.

referral   directing a client to a therapist or other professional who provides treatment. Clients may be referred by another professional, for example a general practitioner (doctor), or may refer themselves. Therapists may refer clients elsewhere if they conclude that they do not have the resources or skills needed to deal with their problems (Steiner's principle of *competency*, see CONTRACT).

reflection (Rogerian person-centred therapy)   the therapist offers back as accurately as possible what the client has presented so that they can look at it objectively, as in a mirror. The therapist may offer back content (what the client has said) and also feeling (inferred empathically from behaviour, tone of voice etc.). Because of its humanistic base, transactional analysis shares many values with the person-centred approach and uses reflection alongside more directive approaches. See Berne's THERAPEUTIC OPERATIONS.

reframing (neurolinguistic programming)   the therapeutic technique of inviting clients to put their concerns imaginatively into a different context or FRAME OF REFERENCE so that they can become aware of aspects that they are missing or DISCOUNTING.

regression   a reversion to an earlier stage of development, usually as a defensive process. An individual who is *in* a Child ego-state is regressed in that he or she is not operating from their current developmental level. However, it is possible to draw on the positive resources of the Child ego-state while retaining access to Adult. In *Transactional Analysis in Psychotherapy* Eric Berne (1961) formulated this as integration of Child material into Adult to produce an INTEGRATED ADULT. A similar process may occur with Parent ego-state material. There are a variety of views among transactional analysts about how to regard the Child ego-state. It may be seen less as a residue of a superseded level of development and more as a repository of valuable qualities that have been lost in later development (a Wordsworthian view: 'the child is father of the man').

Regression may be facilitated as a therapeutic technique. This must be done within a clear CONTRACT and within a structure that provides for adequate physical and emotional safety. Therapeutic interventions while in the regressed state may give access to early issues that would be difficult to work with in other ways, but this type of work raises professional and ethical issues that must be carefully addressed. See REPARENTING.

Reichian based on the work of the post-Freudian analyst Wilhelm Reich. Reich's main theoretical contribution was to the theory of character analysis but the aspect of his work that now receives most attention is the connections that he traced between body states and psychological problems (for example, body armouring) and which he explained in terms of an energy theory (orgone energy). Modern post-Reichian therapies include BIOENERGETICS and Radix. Reich's approach has been introduced into transactional analysis; see BODY SCRIPTING and BODY WORK.

reinforcing memories a memory of a past negative experience that is used to reinforce a SCRIPT BELIEF. There is a tendency to give weight to, and therefore to keep in memory, events that seem to confirm script beliefs, while events that disconfirm them may be easily forgotten. Someone who has a script belief 'I am unlovable' will pay particular attention to circumstances in which they appear to have been rejected and will acquire a large collection of such memories which will reinforce their script belief, while they are likely to find ways of DISCOUNTING disconfirming experiences ('they did not really mean it, they were just being polite'). See RACKET SYSTEM.

reinforcement (behaviourism) associating a reward with a specific behaviour and thus making it more probable that the behaviour will be repeated. This is the basis of operant conditioning and is one of the psychological principles underlying the transactional analysis concept of STROKING.

rejection the experience of not being accepted, invited to feel that one is not wanted or unacceptable (unlovable). Life will inevitably include such experiences but they are particularly damaging in early childhood where they may set up lifelong patterns of expected rejection (which may become a self-fulfilling prophecy) and low self-esteem. Experiences of rejection in childhood are likely to lead to a Don't Exist INJUNCTION.

relationship the pattern of attachment and interaction between two people. From birth onwards human beings exist in relationships and healthy development cannot occur unless the individual is supported, challenged and socialised within a suitable relationship system. Through its power to analyse transactions and map stroking, transactional analysis is able to map relationship processes. Psychological problems are frequently initially failures of relationships. The relationship between the client and the therapist is an important factor in all psychotherapies, including those that accord it little significance (e.g. classical behaviourism). The classical psychodynamic approach sees relationship as important but also threatening to the therapeutic process, which centres on the interpretation of transference. It therefore seeks to control this relationship and restrict the level of contact that this entails. The more relaxed attitude to relationship that transactional analysis adopts derives from its different theoretical position. It finds much of its information in the behaviours (acting out) that are occurring constantly in many contexts and continue to do so even in contactful relationship structures. The relationship is thus set free to become a therapeutic resource, offering some of the qualities that were lacking in the client's original experience. Mary Goulding referred to this approach to therapy as 'corrective closeness'.

repair inevitably, relationships sometimes suffer damage, for example when the mother fails to understand the child's need or responds to her own need at the expense of the child. Analogous processes occur within therapy. In either case when the damage is recognised a repair can be made (Erskine, 1993). The key part of this is the acknowledgement of the damage and its significance to the other.

reparenting providing experiences of parenting to clients in psychotherapy to deal with DEVELOPMENTAL DEFICITS. The approach was originated by the Schiffs who used a radical reparenting technique with extremely disturbed clients. This involved breaking all contact with the original parents, inviting the clients to regress and virtually bringing them up again as a member of the therapist's family. Despite some remarkable results, aspects of this technique were controversial and eventually led to a break between the Schiffs and the transactional analysis movement. Nevertheless the Schiffs were highly influential, founding the Cathexis school, one of the major schools of transactional analysis, and making outstanding contributions to transactional analysis theory. Aaron and Jacqui Schiff received the Eric Berne Memorial Scientific Award in 1974 for their work on passivity and discounting (Schiff and Schiff, 1971). Modified versions of their reparenting methods are used in therapeutic communities by some transactional analysts and much more limited reparenting techniques have been developed that can be incorporated into usual types of therapy where client/therapist contact is limited to an hour each week. These involved working within clear limits agreed within a reparenting contract. See SPOT REPARENTING.

reparenting the Parent a therapeutic technique developed by Mellor and Adrewartha (1980) that involves getting the client to project out the Parent ego-state and working with it to make good developmental deficits by providing good parenting experiences. See also PARENT INTERVIEW.

repetition compulsion (psychoanalysis) a tendency to revert to earlier conditions and thus to resist therapeutic change. Freud originally attributed this to the *death instinct*, a postulated drive to return to the inanimate. This idea possibly influenced some of Berne's and Steiner's more pessimistic theorising about script. Object relations theorists see the resistance to therapeutic change as related to the need to give up attachments to internal objects (introjected others; in transactional analysis terms, Parent ego-state contents). That is, the Child has to abandon its old relationship to the Parent. This involves a process akin to mourning. The term *repetition compulsion* is also used to describe fixed repetitive behaviour patterns, which may represent an attempt to recreate original traumas in order to resolve them (for example, people who repeatedly and unconsciously set up relationships with violent partners). This is one of the dynamics that lie behind the playing of GAMES.

Rescue to do something for someone else in a way that undermines their autonomy. This use of the term is distinguished from legitimate acts of rescue (where the help is really needed) by spelling it with a capital letter. Rescuing involves DISCOUNTING the power of the other person to act effectively and take charge of their own life and the Rescuer comes from an I+U–position (see LIFE POSITIONS). Rescuing involves an invitation into SYMBIOSIS.

Rescuer role (also Rescuer) the DRAMA TRIANGLE role, which involves inviting others into Rescue (the initial capital indicates that a drama triangle role is being referred to and not legitimate rescue). The Rescuer is discounting the supposed Victim's ability to deal with the situation himself or herself and is probably being grandiose about his or her ability to solve the problem.

resolution (1) an intention to act in a particular way (for example, a New Year's resolution). The outcome is likely to depend on the ego-state in which the resolution is made. Resolutions are often made in Child in response to internal pressure from Parent. Usually the Child will quickly find a way of wriggling out of this and there will be no long-term behavioural change.

resolution (2) the solving of a problem or group of problems or release from a state of internal conflict, for example the resolution of an IMPASSE.

responsibility transactional analysis takes the philosophical position that people are responsible for their own lives, thinking, feelings and behaviour. We need to accept limited responsibility for those who are vulnerable or

who are placed (or by agreement place themselves) in our care such as children or clients. Even if we accept some responsibility, we need to encourage the person in our care to be as autonomous as he or she can within the context. Attempts to shift responsibility are usually manipulative. 'I only did it because of you' may be acceptable if there was clear prior agreement but not otherwise. 'You made me angry' implies a responsibility for other people's feelings, however 'I felt angry about what you said' is likely to be a statement of fact. See I STATEMENTS.

review discussion of the therapy process and what has been achieved. The THERAPY CONTRACT may make provision for regular review sessions. Transactional analysis is a contractual process and will include provision for regular review of outstanding contracts.

rituals a form of TIME STRUCTURING in which the transactions follow an agreed pattern so that they are highly predictable. An example is the greeting ritual 'Hello, how are you?' 'OK thanks'. Rituals are safe but yield few strokes.

Rogerian relating to the approach of the American therapist Carl Rogers. This therapeutic method is usually referred to as *client-centred* or *person-centred*. Rogers' original term, non-directive therapy, is no longer used. From a position of unconditional positive regard the therapist facilitates the client in making his or her own evaluation of their situation and life process. Because of its humanistic base transactional analysis shares many values with the person-centred approach but is prepared to utilise more directive approaches. See PERSON-CENTRED COUNSELLING.

role a position in relation to others adopted temporarily or in specific contexts, for example mother, wife, teacher, friend. A role provides only limited opportunity to express the personality and may be highly circumscribed by the expectations of others (role senders), that is playing a role involves not being fully AUTHENTIC. The three positions (Persecutor, Rescuer and Victim) on the DRAMA TRIANGLE are referred to as roles since they are all unauthentic.

rubber band this describes an abrupt move into a Child ego-state so that one finds oneself thinking, feeling and behaving as one did in the past, contacting old beliefs and construing ones experience in the old way. It is as if, as we developed, we remained connected to a point in the past by a rubber band. This stretched as we grew but has suddenly contracted and whisked us back. This term is a description of the experience of being in TRANSFERENCE. It is usually used to refer to negative experiences.

rules of communication these rules predict the outcomes of different types of TRANSACTION (Berne, 1964).

The first rule of communication states that 'so long as transactions remain complementary communication *can* continue indefinitely'. COMPLEMENTARY TRANSACTION means that the ego-state that replies is the one that was addressed, and the reply is directed to the ego-state that initiated (i.e. both parties are agreed as to who should be in which ego-state). An example would be a stimulus Parent to Child responded to by Child to Parent. When illustrated, the vectors of a complementary transaction run parallel.

The second rule of communication states that 'when a transaction is crossed a break in communication results and one or both individuals will need to shift ego-states in order for communication to be re-established.' A CROSSED TRANSACTION occurs when the ego-state that answers is not the one that was addressed, i.e. the parties disagree as to who should be in which ego-state. An example would be a transaction Adult to Adult responded to Parent to Child. When illustrated the vectors usually do not run parallel and often cross.

The third rule of communication states that 'the behavioural outcome of an ULTERIOR TRANSACTION is determined at the psychological and not at the social level'. An ulterior transaction operates at two levels simultaneously. There is a *social transaction* that is the ostensible meaning of the transaction and is usually the literal meaning of the words spoken. This meaning is socially acceptable. There is also a second meaning that is understood by both participants. This understanding may not be fully in awareness and certainly will not be acknowledged. This is the psychological level transaction whose content is often not socially acceptable.

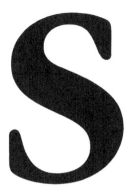

sabotage behaviours or thought patterns that undermine the therapy process. This is indicative of internal conflict, the sabotage often being due to the Child ego-state hanging on to an old and well-tried defensive strategy.

SAD see SEASONAL AFFECTIVE DISORDER.

sadness one of the FOUR AUTHENTIC FEELINGS, sadness is experienced in the process of mourning. It relates to the loss of someone or something one has been attached to and expressing the feeling and having it validated by others helps in the process of letting go so that new attachments can be made. Unlike other authentic feelings, its time frame is the past. Although it is classified as an authentic feeling, it can be expressed unauthentically as a RACKET FEELING. Sadness should be distinguished from UNHAPPINESS and DEPRESSION.

Santa Claus, waiting for passively waiting for some imagined future good outcome, especially as a long-term strategy in SCRIPT.

Schiff, Aaron with Jacqui Lee Schiff jointly received the Eric Berne Memorial Scientific Award in 1974 for work on passivity and the four discounts (Schiff and Schiff, 1971).

Schiff, Jacqui Lee transactional analyst. She has made major contributions to theory and practice and, with Aaron Schiff, was awarded the Eric Berne Memorial Prize in 1974 for her work on passivity and the four discounts. She founded the Cathexis Institute which gave its name to the Cathexis school of transactional analysis. Her major innovation was the technique of REPARENTING, which she claimed was able to cure schizophrenia. As originally practised, this involved inviting the client to regress to a childhood state and bringing him or her up again within the therapist's 'family' or therapeutic community. Within this supportive environment there was high confrontation of dysfunctional behaviours. It was therefore a highly interventionist approach with a strong emphasis on behaviour. The level of intervention that Jacqui Schiff was using with her clients caused concern within the transactional analysis community where some felt it breached the principle of 'I'm OK, You're OK'. This disagreement eventually led to a breach between her and the transactional analysis community although the Cathexis school within transactional analysis remains active and influential.

Schiffian theory the body of transactional analysis theory developed by Jacqui

Lee Schiff and her co-workers. This centres around the therapeutic use of REPARENTING. Important concepts include the FOUR PASSIVE BEHAVIOURS, SYMBIOSIS, DISCOUNTING, the DISCOUNT MATRIX, REDEFINING and FRAME OF REFERENCE. This constitutes one of the major theoretical areas of transactional analysis, which is usually referred to as the Cathexis school (the Schiffs called their organisation the Cathexis Institute). The major source of information on this approach is *The Cathexis Reader: Transactional Analysis Treatment of Psychosis* (Schiff et al., 1975).

schizoid personality adaptation a pattern of personality organisation characterised by passivity, withdrawal and a separation of feeling and thinking. The schizoid client has suffered a failure in contact by the caretaker in early childhood resulting in withdrawal and getting needs met in fantasy. Often there was SECOND-ORDER SYMBIOSIS with the mother. They usually have a rich fantasy life so may be highly creative. Their WARE SEQUENCE is behaviour (passive), thinking, feeling, so feeling is doubly defended. Feelings are often dealt with mainly in fantasy (for example, writing love poems instead of relating to a partner).

schizophrenia a serious mental illness characterised by acute psychotic episodes and disturbances of thought and perception. It is uncertain how far it is caused by psychological factors or disturbances of brain biochemistry. Both may be involved. The concept of schizophrenia has been criticised for being over-inclusive and in fact may signify a group of disorders. The SCHIFFS (Cathexis school) treated schizophrenics using a radical REPARENTING approach for which they claimed a high level of success. See Schiff and Day (1970).

Schlemiel a game described by Berne (1964) in which the player repeatedly makes 'messes' (problems for others) and then apologises and seeks to be forgiven. As described it does not meet all the criteria of Berne's later (1972) definitions of a game.

schools of transactional analysis there are three major schools:

- the CLASSICAL SCHOOL, representing the work of Berne and those closely associated with him (e.g. Steiner);
- the REDECISION SCHOOL, based on the work of Robert and Mary Goulding;
- the CATHEXIS (or Schiffian) school based on the work of Jacqui Schiff and co-workers. See separate entries.

A new school is emerging that seeks to integrate transactional analysis with certain aspects of psychoanalytic thinking. This is associated with transactional analysts such as Moiso and Erskine. Stewart (1996a) has suggested the name 'psychoanalytic renaissance' for this.

script an unconscious life pattern based on early decisions made, usually out of awareness, in childhood. This may take many years or even a lifetime to run its course. The final outcome resulting from the script process (e.g. isolation) is called the PAYOFF. This is also considered to arise from early decisions. The term payoff suggests that this endpoint in some ways solves a life problem in accordance with the logic of the Child and that this 'solution' acts as a motivator (script moves towards the payoff, which is a teleological view) or that the payoff brings other benefits (see SECONDARY GAIN). An alternative formulation is to see script as representing a TRANSFERENTIAL replay of unresolved life issues, the drama being cast from people currently available who transferentially represent significant figures in the past. It is possible for issues to be worked through in this way but usually the amount of DISCOUNTING of current reality and PROJECTING of issues from the past results in a replay of the original outcome thus reinforcing script.

There has been debate as to whether there can be a positive script. Unconscious patterns may be useful but will always suffer the disadvantage that they cannot readily be changed to adjust to current reality. Essentially all script behaviours involve discounting. Stewart and Joines (1987) define script as that part of the FRAME OF REFERENCE that involves discounting. See SCRIPT APPARATUS, SCRIPT MATRIX, SCRIPT SYSTEM, PROCESS SCRIPT, EARLY LIFE DECISION.

script apparatus the elements which make up the script. These include INJUNCTIONS, COUNTERINJUNCTIONS, PROGRAM, PERMISSIONS AND EARLY LIFE DECISIONS.

script backlash after a movement out of script the client may experience a severe reaction of anxiety, guilt etc. This may be seen in terms of the Parent punishing the Child for its transgression. It is important that sufficient PROTECTION is available from the therapist to deal with this if it occurs.

script belief a belief about self, others or the world arrived at in childhood in an attempt to deal with unfinished business (usually feelings that have not been appropriately responded to) by 'explaining away' (making cognitive closure). Script beliefs are an important element in the SCRIPT (RACKET) system of Erskine and Zalcman (1979).

script diagrams the two main ways of illustrating the script are Steiner's SCRIPT MATRIX and the RACKET SYSTEM (sometimes called the SCRIPT SYSTEM) of Erskine and Zalcman (1979).

script matrix a diagram showing how a client received his or her INJUNCTIONS, COUNTERINJUNCTIONS and PROGRAM MESSAGES from parents' ego-states. In Steiner's (1966) original model the script is shown as held in all three ego-states of the client. Woollams and Brown (1978) hold that the script is held in the Child and is distributed between the three second-order ego-states P_1, A_1 and C_1.

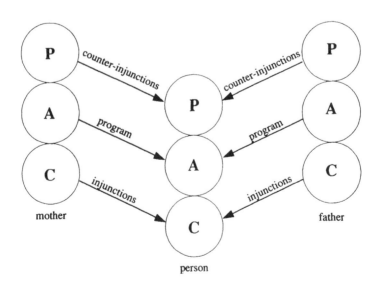

Figure 23 Script matrix — Steiner (Steiner, 1966).

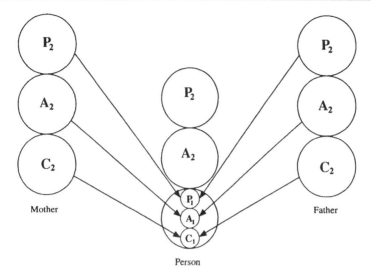

Figure 24 Script matrix — Woollams and Brown (Woollams and Brown, 1978).

script payoff SEE PAYOFF.

script process the way the script is lived out. This tends to follow one of a small number of characteristic patterns. See PROCESS SCRIPT.

script proper the part of the script specified by INJUNCTIONS. This represents the underlying psychological damage that drives script behaviour. However, the way in which the script is worked out in behaviours is heavily influenced by the COUNTERSCRIPT, which is specified by the COUNTERINJUNCTIONS.

script questionnaire a set of questions designed to elicit information on script. See examples in Berne (1972).

script sign a behaviour which indicates that a person is in their script. This is often a characteristic gesture, expression posture or movement of some kind but also includes words, paralinguistic signals such as tone of voice and even bodily states such as headaches. (Also called *script signal.*)

script system an alternative name for the RACKET SYSTEM.

script, types of scripts may be winning (achieving the specified objective), non-winning (banal) or losing. Steiner (1974) classified scripts as loveless, joyless and mindless according to their central theme. Scripts are also classified according to the degree of payoff (first, second or third-degree). A losing script with a third degree (tragic) payoff is known as a *hamartic* script. Scripts are also classified according to their process types. See PROCESS SCRIPT, SCRIPT PROPER.

scriptbound limited by SCRIPT. The name given by Adrienne Lee to her diagrammatic presentation of script. See DROWNING PERSON DIAGRAM.

sculpting a technique in which the client is invited to generate a pattern in the environment that symbolises their internal state. In a group this may involve getting the group members to arrange themselves in a pattern and in postures that symbolise the client's feelings about them (their distance, their warmth or threatening quality) or about members of the client's family of origin or other important others that they represent. The configuration may then be worked on by asking them to change position. Inanimate objects can be used in the same way. This technique enables unacknowledged (unconscious) thoughts and feelings to be projected and then dealt with symbolically. This technique, which is essentially a development of PSYCHO-DRAMA, is often employed by transactional analysts and facilitates contact with the Child ego-state.

seasonal affective disorder (SAD) a type of depression that occurs during winter and is believed to be associated with lack of exposure to daylight. Treatment by exposure to artificial daylight is claimed to help sufferers. Depression may have multiple causes, so a diagnosis of SAD should not preclude the use of a psychotherapeutic approach such as transactional analysis.

second-order analysis of ego-states see EGO-STATE, SECOND-ORDER ANALYSIS.

second-order structural analysis see EGO-STATE, SECOND-ORDER ANALYSIS.

second-order symbiosis see SYMBIOSIS, SECOND ORDER.

second rule of communication Berne (1964) stated three rules of communication that predict the outcome of transactions. The second rule states that when a communication is crossed, a break in communication results and one or both individuals will need to shift ego-states in order for communications to be re-established. *Crossed* means that the answer was received from an ego-state other than the one addressed; that is, the parties cannot agree on who is to be in which ego-state. When illustrated, this situation usually results in crossed vectors. Communication is not possible until there is such agreement although sometimes the parties continue to talk

at each other, although not *to* each other. See RULES OF COMMUNICATION

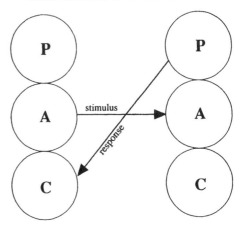

Figure 25 A crossed transaction.

secondary gain psychological or social benefit obtained from a symptom or problem, for example by inviting a partner into a caregiving (symbiotic) role as in the GAME of WOODEN LEG. See also PAYOFF, CODEPENDENCY, SYMBIOSIS.

secondary process (psychoanalysis) thinking that is logical and based on reality. This is characteristic of the Adult ego-state whereas PRIMARY PROCESS is more characteristic of the Child. See also MAGICAL THINKING.

See How Hard I Tried a GAME initiated from the VICTIM position, which seeks to create and sustain symbiosis by ineffective struggling with a problem.

See What You Made Me Do a GAME in which the initiator, from the VICTIM position, seeks to create symbiosis by getting others to take responsibility for his or her actions.

self the person as he or she experiences himself or herself, as having a distinctive identity, able to initiate actions and as being perceived by and reacted to by others. Structures such as the ego in psychoanalysis or one of the ego-states in transactional analysis do not correspond to the self although they provide descriptions of a part of the psychic apparatus where the experience of selfhood is manifested. The concept of self is subjective (phenomenological) whereas these are objective descriptions. Berne (1961) pointed out that there may be a separation between that which is (the self) and that which acts (the executive). In this case the self may perceive the action as out of character and alien (EGO DYSTONIC). Berne explained this in terms of the distribution of different types of ENERGY between the ego-states.

self-esteem positive self-valuation. This is enhanced by being valued (receiving positive STROKING, especially unconditional stroking, that is stroking for being). It is damaged by unjust criticism, the negative projections of others and being ignored. Low self-esteem is usually associated with a belief, often rooted in childhood experiences, that the person has only a conditional right to exist and be himself or herself (Don't Exist, Don't Be You and Don't Be Important INJUNCTIONS defended by COMPOUND DECISIONS). For a transactional analysis approach to working with self-esteem issues, see Clark (1978).

self-fulfilling prophecy action in relation to an imagined future outcome that makes the outcome more probable (e.g. being hostile to people who we fear may reject us).

self-harm damage to the body. This may include SUBSTANCE ABUSE, SELF-MUTILATION and SUICIDE. Self-harm is one of the three ESCAPE HATCHES.

self-mutilation this commonly takes the form of cutting the arms and is often seen in seriously disturbed clients. It is likely to indicate a powerful Don't Exist injunction. At its most serious level body parts may be cut off (e.g. Van Gogh's ear).

self-regard see SELF-ESTEEM.

self-reparenting a method developed by the transactional analyst Muriel James (1974), for which she received the Eric Berne Memorial Scientific Award in 1983. The method involves generating new Parent content to supplement or replace existing defective Parent. The Adult is actively involved in doing this for the self, drawing on internal sources such as ideas, decisions, memories of positive Parent figures, etc. This can be done with the guidance of the therapist but the therapist does not take on the parent role as in the other forms of REPARENTING.

self-sabotage acting, usually in therapy and out of awareness, to undermine one's own endeavours. The SCRIPT has been elaborated in the Child ego-state in an attempt to make his or her world safe and satisfy STROKING needs. It therefore has a defensive function although it is in fact damaging as it is based on misinformation, archaic information or a confused understanding of reality. However, to the Child ego-state it is essential for safety or even survival. Psychotherapy, by challenging the script, makes the Child feel unsafe and so tends to set up internal conflict that may lead to self-sabotage. See also IMPASSE.

self-talk sub-vocal or inaudible statements made to the self that influence behaviour. From a transactional analysis standpoint this may be regarded as an intervention in the INTERNAL DIALOGUE between ego-states, the voicing of one of the participants serving to reinforce it. Positively, the self-talk may represent Adult thinking or Parent support or information. However, it may be a negative Parent voice ('you've done it again!'). Self-talk can also be used actively, e.g. giving oneself AFFIRMATIONS.

separation anxiety anxiety derived originally from interruption in the caregiver's contact with the child, which interfered with the baby's attachment to the mother or caregiver and consequently its sense of security. In Bowlby's (1969) view this forms the basis for all later anxieties relating to separations.

Sex in Human Loving this book by Eric Berne was published in the year of his death (1970). In his characteristic lucid, humorous and incisive style he looks at human sexual relationships in terms of transactional analysis theory.

shame self-judgement for some public display of inadequacy or immorality and the emotional state that accompanies this. There is a social dimension to shame that may be lacking in guilt; it involves the imagined condemnation of an audience. Shaming is often used by parents to control children and in the experience of shame the Parent ego-state is attacking the Child in the INTERNAL DIALOGUE in a way that often closely parallels the original family process. In accepting shaming the child is colluding in the parents' process of negative projection in an attempt to obtain love. Shame undermines the individual and does not support positive change, so it is regarded as a RACKET FEELING. See Erskine (1994), English (1994) and Cornell (1994).

'should' statements a statement implying a moral imperative to act in a certain way. This usually indicates that the Parent ego-state is active.

Sigmund, Eric received an Eric Berne Memorial Scientific Award jointly with Ken Mellor in 1980 for his work on DISCOUNTING and REDEFINING (Mellor and Sigmund 1975a, 1975b).

social anxiety anxiety experienced in social situations associated with feelings of shyness and embarrassment.

social control a stage early in therapy in which sufficient insight has been achieved for inappropriate behaviours to be identified and avoided and more appropriate behaviours chosen. This will occur when substantial DECONTAMINATION of Adult has been achieved, however no changes will have occurred in Child or Parent so symptoms will not have been relieved. See STAGES OF THERAPY.

social level the manifest message of an ulterior transaction (what appears to be being said) is the social level message. A second message is being transmitted at the psychological level and it is this that decides the outcome of the transaction. See TRANSACTION, ULTERIOR.

social psychiatry Eric Berne chose the title San Francisco Social Psychiatry Seminars for the meeting of professionals that took place at his home every Tuesday evening from 1958. Here many of the ideas of transactional analysis were burnished and developed. The term 'social psychiatry' derives from Harry Stack Sullivan (1953) who was one of the first people to place psychiatric problems in a social psychological framework, as being located not solely in the individual but also in his or her relationship with society. A one-person psychology such as drive theory psychoanalysis ignores an important part of the system. Transactional analysis, with its ability to conceptualise and analyse *transactions* between individuals is ideally equipped to develop this approach.

soft closure SEE ESCAPE HATCHES.

somatic relating to the body. See also PSYCHOSOMATIC.

somatic Child the Child in the Child ego-state or C_1. So called because the young child experiences the world mainly through body sensations. Disturbances at this level may manifest via the body (e.g. through PSYCHOSOMATIC illness).

somatise to convert a psychological symptom into a body state as occurs in PSYCHOSOMATIC illness (e.g. anxiety being expressed as eczema). This involves the Child in the Child ego-state or SOMATIC CHILD C₁.

special fields a specific area of application of transactional analysis. The Certified Transactional Analyst examination can be taken in each of four special fields: clinical, educational, organisational and counselling.

specification see THERAPEUTIC OPERATIONS.

splitting (Kleinian psychoanalysis) a state in which there is a lack of integration between parts of the psyche. Multiple personality disorder (MPD) represents an extreme state but there is evidence for some degree of splitting in many people and few people experience themselves at all times as fully integrated. Transactional analysis, with its division of the ego into three ego-states, is a model of a split ego. Berne (1961) saw this as ultimately developing into a single structure, the integrated Adult. Kleinians regard splitting as a very early defence that is employed by the baby to deal with its inconsistent experience of the mother (good breast and bad breast) until it has the mental resources to deal with ambivalence and can see the mother as one person who is loving, although she sometimes fails to meet the child's needs (the child achieves OBJECT CONSTANCY). This early splitting is reflected in the transactional analysis model of the splitting of the Parent in the Child ego-state (P₁) into good and bad parts (often called the Fairy Godmother and the Pig Parent or ogre).

spontaneity the ability to react genuinely and without inhibitions in the moment. This is characteristic of the natural Child (free Child). ADAPTATION to the parents or others results in loss of spontaneity.

spot reparenting a technique for limited REPARENTING that can be used in ordinary weekly therapy (c.f. Schiffian reparenting, which requires prolonged and intensive involvement between the therapist and client). The technique was developed by Osnes (1974) and involves the client regressing to a traumatic experience and receiving positive parenting from the therapist. The intervention is focused on a specific point in the client's experience, just as a laser might be used in medical treatment.

stages of therapy Berne (1961, 1972) suggested that psychotherapy moves through four stages of 'cure'.

1. The client has achieved sufficient insight into his or her script to take control of his or her behaviour and avoid many scripty behaviours, however the script mechanism is still intact. The client takes control from Adult although Child and Parent are unchanged. Berne called this stage *social control* and as the Adult often finds itself in opposition to the pull of the Child and Parent it requires a considerable expenditure of energy by the Adult to maintain it.
2. In the next stage the client has started to make changes in the Child and Parent ego-states. As a result, they experience less internal pressure to engage in scripty behaviour and less energy is required to stay out of script. He called this stage *symptomatic relief*.
3. In the third stage the client has taken in (introjected) the therapist as a substitute for his or her original parent. As the new parent gives more positive messages than the old one they find it easier to stay out of script. Berne called this stage *transference*

115

cure. It will remain stable as long as the client can keep the therapist around in his or her head, certainly for the duration of therapy and perhaps beyond if the new parent can be as firmly retained as the old one. However, there is the risk of lapsing back into script.

4. In the fourth and final stage the client is assisted in making fundamental changes in the Child egostate with Adult support. The client is thus able to move permanently out of script. In his earlier writing Berne called this *psychoanalytic cure* but later, with the development of life script theory, he renamed it *script cure*.

There are a number of other systems for describing the stages of therapeutic change, notably those of Erskine (1973) and Woollams and Brown (1978).

stamps (also trading stamps) feelings that are held so that they can be used to manipulate others. Stamps are collected by indulging in RACKET BEHAVIOURS that invite others into treating us in a certain way (e.g. inviting us into anger so that we can collect an anger stamp). Stamps are later used to achieve a scripty outcome, which the collected stamps 'justify'. This is called 'cashing in the stamps', for example a collection of resentment stamps can be cashed in for a row with one's partner.

standards of practice major counselling and psychotherapy organisations such as ITA (the Institute for Transactional Analysis), EATA (the European Association for Transactional Analysis), ITAA (the International Transactional Analysis Association) and BAC (the British Association for Counselling) have codes of professional practice in addition to, or in association with, their ethical codes. These provide guidelines on matters such as competence, professional development, con-

tracting and the way counsellors represents themselves and what they can offer, both within the therapeutic relationship and in advertising. See Appendix 3.

Steiner, Claude transactional analyst. A close associate of Eric Berne, Claude Steiner had a major influence on the development of transactional analysis and his work is included in the Classic School. He is best known for developing script theory, in particular the SCRIPT MATRIX. Other important contributions to transactional analysis include his work on CONTRACTING and the STROKE ECONOMY. He was given Eric Berne Memorial Scientific Awards in 1971 (script matrix) and again in 1980 (stroke economy). He is the author of a number of important books and articles on transactional analysis including *Games Alcoholics Play* (1971) and *Scripts People Live* (1974).

stimulus hunger the need for mental and physical stimulation. Such stimulation appears to be essential for the normal development and psychological health of all mammals. Eric Berne (1964) suggested that in human beings this is manifested primarily as a hunger for recognition by others (RECOGNITION HUNGER). He called acts of recognition STROKES since in infants these are often tactile.

stopper in the MINISCRIPT the position shifted to when the defence provided by a DRIVER against an INJUNCTION fails so that the injunction is responded to. This results in a shift from the position of conditional OKness achieved with the driver (I'm OK *if* . . .) to an I–U+ LIFE POSITION.

storming the third stage in Tuckman's (1965, Tuckman and Jensen, 1977) classification of the stages of small group development. The complete sequence is 'forming', 'norming', 'storming' and performing. A further stage in which the group focuses on its termination has been called 'mourning' by Lacousiere (1980). Clarkson (1992) has integrated Tuckman's theories with those of Berne (1963, 1966). She identifies Tuckman's storming stage with Berne's adapted group imago. See STAGES OF GROUP DEVELOPMENT.

story telling allowing the client to tell his or her story is an important part of psychotherapy, giving valuable script information and helping the client to feel heard and validated by the therapist. Although it is important for the client to feel heard, exhaustive story telling is likely to mean that the therapist and client are playing the GAME of Archeology. See FLIGHT INTO HISTORY. One way of constraining the process of telling the life history is to use a SCRIPT QUESTIONNAIRE. Imaginative story telling, in which the client is invited to make up a story, can be used to access script (unconscious) material that will be expressed symbolically. Therapeutic interventions can be made at the symbolic level by inviting the client to change the story. Another approach is for the client and therapist to create the story jointly, the therapist making a therapeutic response to what the client presents while remaining within the symbolic frame of the story.

strategy in transactional analysis TREATMENT PLANNING. This term signifies a plan for achieving a therapeutic objective.

stress a situation in which an increased demand is being placed on the adjustment systems of the person. Stress that does not exceed an individual's adjustment capacity will not be harmful and may even be perceived as pleasantly stimulating because it satisfies STIMULUS HUNGER. Stress may be due to external circumstances (e.g.

losing one's job) or internal (e.g. psychological or physical problems) and the response to stress may occur at either or both levels (e.g. an external stressor may result in depression and eczema).

stress scale Woollams and Brown (1978) developed a scale for expressing levels of psychological stress. They suggest that REDECISIONS are rarely complete but can be seen in terms of the protection that they offer against a script element such as an INJUNCTION becoming active under stress. The more profound the redecision the greater will be the level of stress necessary before the injunction will become active.

stroke a unit of recognition, so called because the human infant first received this mainly through touch. A stroke can be a smile, a phrase of praise or criticism or another of the numerous social signals which humans give each other. Strokes can be positive ('well done'), negative ('you loused that up'), conditional ('I like you when you smile like that') or unconditional ('I hate you'). They can also be verbal or non-verbal. Combining these three categories, there are eight types of stroke.

stroke bank positive strokes (such as praise) can be stored in memory and recalled when stroke deprived. This is called using a stroke bank.

stroke economy Steiner (1974) suggested that cultural patterns encourage parents to create a stroke shortage for children. This raises the value of the strokes they supply and therefore makes the children more controllable. He saw this shortage economy as being sustained through five restrictive rules about stroking:

• Don't give strokes when you have them to give.

- Don't ask for strokes when you need them.
- Don't accept strokes if you want them.
- Don't reject strokes when you don't want them.
- Don't give yourself strokes.

Steiner (1974) expresses this message imaginatively through a fairy story 'A Fuzzy Tale'. See WARM FUZZIES, COLD PRICK-LIES.

stroke filter the elimination or distortion of strokes that are 'surplus to requirements' because they exceed those allowed by the STROKE QUOTIENT.

stroke quotient early experiences result in an expected ratio between positive and negative strokes received. For example, this might be four negative strokes to one positive. This ratio is the stroke quotient. Any disturbance in the stroke quotient is likely to be resisted. Surplus strokes may be eliminated (DIS-COUNTED) or even changed from positive to negative: 'she did not really mean those nice things, she was just being patronising because she despises me'. This is called using the STROKE FILTER.

stroking giving strokes (units of recognition). See STROKE.

stroking profile a diagram in the form of a bar chart that illustrates an individual's habitual patterns for dealing with strokes, i.e. the tendency for positive and negative, unconditional and conditional strokes to be asked for, accepted or refused.

structural analysis analysis of ego in terms of intrapsychic structures. First-order structural analysis shows three intrapsychic structures: the Parent, Adult and Child ego-states. Second-order structural analysis shows the presence of subsidiary, historically earlier, ego-states within the Parent and Child ego-states. Functional analysis shows the functions associated with each ego-state and does not suggest that each function is associated with a structural element, its conceptual framework being behavioural rather than intrapsychic. See EGO-STATES, SEC-OND-ORDER ANALYSIS OF EGO-STATES.

structural model of ego-states see STRUCTURAL ANALYSIS.

structure the way in which something is constructed. The ego-state theory postulates intrapsychic structures and relates these to observable behaviours. Psychoanalytic theory with its concepts of mental organs (id, ego and super-ego) and zones of differential awareness and accessibility (conscious, pre-conscious and unconscious) is likewise a structural theory.

structure hunger Berne (1964) concluded that there is a basic need for the structuring of time that manifests as structure hunger. This is one of the factors motivating interpersonal transactions and results in the development of characteristic patterns of structuring time. He identified six patterns of time structuring:

withdrawal
rituals
pastimes
activities
games
intimacy
See individual entries.

Stuntz multiple chair work (five chair work) Stuntz (1973) described a multiple chair technique. Each of the five FUNCTIONAL EGO-STATES (controlling Parent, nurturant Parent, Adult, adapted Child, free Child) is allocated a chair. The client is invited to move between the chairs speaking from the relevant ego-state. This sets up a dialogue between ego-states to elucidate and resolve internal conflict.

Stupid a GAME in which individuals obtain strokes by inviting others to think for them and criticise them thus the initiator of the game is able to achieve SYMBIOSIS from a Child position.

subconscious the part of the mind that contains material that is not currently conscious. It often signifies that part of the mind that, although not currently conscious, can become so, thus corresponding to the Freudian concept of the preconscious. Transactional analysts may also use these terms but usually prefer to talk of psychological material being in or out of awareness, using a metaphor of a *process*, awareness, which is necessary for consciousness, rather than a *place* in the mind (subconscious, unconscious) from which material must be retrieved.

subjectivity the state of being a subject relating to others or OBJECTS from a unique personal viewpoint. Our own personal world of experiences, feelings and ideas. This is more real to us (that is it impinges on us more strongly) than the experiences of others or statements about what is held to be objectively real (e.g. scientific knowledge). We need to be in touch with our own subjective world but to withdraw too far into it would be to lose contact with the world we share with others and which impinges on our own bodies, which are a part of that external world. Psychosis represents the extreme point of such withdrawal. Transactional analysis aims to be a two-person psychology that can integrate the subjective and objective views through its understanding of the connections between observable behaviours (e.g. SCRIPT SIGNS, behavioural manifestations of ego-states) and subjective mental processes. See also INTERSUBJECTIVITY.

sub-personality a semi-autonomous part of the personality resulting from the use of the defence of DISSOCIATION.

Some degree of splitting into discrete intrapsychic structures (e.g. ego-states) is universal. The term sub-personality is usually reserved for situations in which the splitting is marked. Accounts of multiple personality disorder (MPD) suggest that this represents an extreme condition in which sub-personalities are so deeply split that they manifest separately and sometimes seem to be unaware of each other's existence.

substance abuse the misuse of chemical substances such as alcohol or non-prescribed drugs to produce psychological changes. Like psychological defences, drugs are used to control anxiety arising from unresolved internal conflicts. Drug misuse therefore constitutes a manifestation of SCRIPT. Steiner (1971) writes about the significance of GAMES in maintaining substance misuse by alcoholics.

suicide killing oneself. One of the three ESCAPE HATCHES. Suicide results when a Don't Exist INJUNCTION is insufficiently defended. This defence may be at two levels: (1) by a counterinjunction such as Please Others leading to a compound decision 'I can exist as long as I please others'; (2) by another injunction such as 'Don't Be Close' leading to the compound decision 'I can exist as long as I don't get close'. These defences may be disturbed by outside events (e.g. a Please Others driver may cease to provide protection if the client experiences a relationship failure and so feels that they are failing to please a significant other). The defences may also be disturbed by intrapsychic change; therapy itself may disturb the defensive system, so adequate PROTECTION must be provided for the client before major change is initiated and this must include escape-hatch closure.

superego (psychoanalysis) an intrapsychic structure (mental organ) that reg-

119

ulates and criticises the ego. In Freud's original formulation the ego is in the unenviable position of having to satisfy the demands of the ID, placate the superego and also deal with the constraints of exterior reality. Transactional analysis sees the functions of the superego as manifesting through the Parent ego-state. This contains introjects of specific parent figures that have been experienced by the client. An objection to this view is that the internal Parent sometimes manifests as more critical and punishing than any historical parent figure. This is explained in terms of two Parent ego-states. An earlier version is within the Child ego-state (P_1) and is largely the creation of child PHANTASY and also incorporates early experiences in which the child saw the parent as enormously powerful (magical Parent) and potentially threatening. This early Parent may be split into idealised and negative forms, sometimes referred to as the Fairy Godmother and the Pig or Witch Parents. This theoretical position is reminiscent of the Kleinian view. Unlike the superego, the Parent ego-state may contain positive and supportive as well as critical aspects of the historical parent. See also SPLITTING.

supervision it is important for both the counsellor or therapist and the client that the professional regularly takes his or her work to supervision and this is a requirement for trainees preparing for the Certified Transactional Analysis examination. This may be with someone of a similar level of training and experience or, more usually, with a more experienced colleague. PEER SUPERVISION cannot be counted towards trainees' supervision requirements. Supervision involves discussion of the therapist's work, possibly illustrated by tapes, to monitor professional and ethical issues as well as personal issues affecting the therapist, which may be influencing the process. The supervi-

sor will also be concerned with the effectiveness of the therapist's work, use of theory and specific difficulties he or she has encountered, as well as his or her professional development. The process provides protection for the client and also for the professional position of the therapist.

sweatshirt self presentation. People behave as if they were wearing sweatshirts with messages on the front and back. The message on the front is the way the person habitually presents himself or herself while on the back is the underlying psychological message. Thus someone who avoids longed for contact because they fear rejection might have on the front 'keep your distance' and on the back 'but don't leave me'.

switch the point in a GAME at which DRAMA TRIANGLE positions are switched. See FORMULA G.

symbiosis (Cathexis school) Symbiosis occurs when two individuals behave as through they constituted a single person. Each person in a symbiosis is DISCOUNTING certain ego-states so that only one Parent, Adult and Child ego state is functioning in the combination.

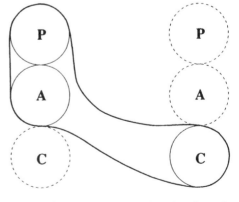

Figure 26 Symbiosis – dotted circles show discounted ego-state.

symbiosis, healthy the normal situation in child care in which the child is able to make use of the resources of the Adult and Parent ego-states of the carer. The degree to which symbiosis is offered needs to be related to the child's growing powers. Parents may DISCOUNT these powers leading to a symbiotic relationship that impedes development.

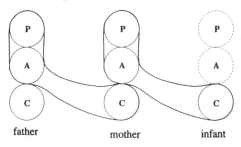

father   mother   infant

Figure 27 First order symbiosis (Schiff et al., 1975).

symbiosis, second order a form of symbiosis (parent/child supportive relationship) in which the parent cares for the child at the social level while the child cares for the parent at the psychological level. In symbiosis the parent cares for the child by drawing on the resources of his or her own Parent and Adult egostates. This makes good the child's deficiencies as it does not yet have these states fully developed. This primary symbiotic relation is usually mainly between the mother and the child. It leaves the mother's Child ego-state unsupported. Ideally the father provides this support to form what Donald Winnicott called the NURSING TRIAD. If this support is not available the mother may turn to the child for support. In doing this she invites the child's developing Parent and Adult, P_1 and A_1, to care for her somatic Child C_1. This leaves the child's own C_1 unsupported. Normal symbiosis is a normal phase of development. Pathological forms of symbiosis, such as second order symbiosis, may become lifelong patterns.

symbiotic invitation a transaction, particularly in therapy, which invites the

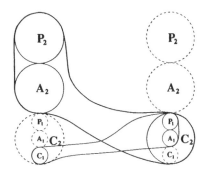

Figure 28 Second order symbiosis (Schiff et al., 1975).

other into a symbiotic (i.e. Child or Parent) position. For example a therapist who adopts a unduly nurturant style or Rescues invites the client into Child. Likewise passive or tentative behaviour may invite the other to enter symbiosis from the Parent position. Symbiotic invitations are not necessarily contraindicated in therapy but their use should be based on clear psychotherapeutic objectives. See SYMBIOSIS.

symptomatic control the stage of transactional analysis psychotherapy in which the client has insight into his or her SYMPTOMS and a reduction of pressure from Child and Parent makes it easier for Adult to maintain control. There is usually an immediate improvement in relationships and the client may consider himself or herself cured; however, although DECONTAMINATION has been achieved, enabling the client to distinguish Child and Parent material from Adult, the Child remains confused and the client has to divert much energy into maintaining control in the face of Child anxiety and Parent pressure. See also STAGES OF THERAPY.

symptom a characteristic sign or indication of a state or disease.

syndrome a group of symptoms characteristically occurring together. PERSONALITY ADAPTATION represents a syndrome approach to diagnosis.

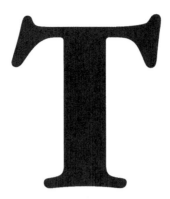

TA 101 the official introduction to transactional analysis, following a syllabus specified by the International Transactional Analysis Association (ITAA). This is usually taught as a two-day intensive workshop although it is also possible to qualify by taking a written examination. Completion of a TA 101 is a requirement for regular membership of the Institute of Transactional Analysis (ITA) and for official transactional analysis training.

tangential transaction see TRANSACTION, TANGENTIAL.

tape recording therapists and counsellors sometimes make tape recordings of sessions with their clients' permission. These enable the processes occurring to be analysed in detail, e.g. it enables them to carry out TRANSACTIONAL ANALYSIS PROPER, and are particularly valuable in the training of psychotherapists and counsellors. Tape recording has a second meaning in transactional analysis, standing figuratively for parental messages that determine script. 'Parent tapes' are 'played back in the head', thus triggering scripty thinking, feeling and behaviour.

technique the specific means and procedures used to carry out therapy, such as script analysis or CUSHION WORK, as opposed to theory, such as the theory of ego-states, which is the system of meaning which guides the use of techniques. Each system of psychotherapy has its own techniques while many techniques are common to the field or large sections of it.

termination ending therapy or counselling. Berne (1961) listed three types of termination: accidental, resistant and therapeutic. Accidental termination occurs when the client moves away or has to terminate because of some external force over which he or she has no control. In resistant termination, which is usually based on fear, dissatisfaction or triumph, there is a plausible excuse or a sudden withdrawal and this indicates that the therapist has overlooked something. The movement to therapeutic termination will be marked by the achievement of contracts and when it is achieved both client and therapist will agree that therapeutic goals have been achieved. Termination will usually involve a final phase of integration and consolidation of gains. Clients sometimes seek to terminate prematurely when the stage of SOCIAL CONTROL is reached. See FLIGHT INTO HEALTH.

terminology of transactional analysis see LANGUAGE OF TRANSACTIONAL ANALYSIS.

TEW see TRAINING ENDORSEMENT WORKSHOP.

Thanatos (psychoanalysis) the death instinct. Referred to by Berne (1957) and possibly an influence on his more pessimistic thinking about SCRIPT. See LIBIDO.

The Mind in Action Eric Berne's first book (Berne, 1947) offering an accessible approach to psychoanalytic theory. The seeds of transactional analysis were beginning to sprout but this was not yet a book on transactional analysis. It was subsequently reissued in an expanded and revised form and incorporating a substantial amount of transactional analysis under the title A LAYMAN'S GUIDE TO PSYCHIATRY AND PSYCHOANALYSIS (Berne, 1957). A further revised edition was published under the same title with contributions from other transactional analysts (Berne, 1967).

The Structure and Dynamics of Organizations and Groups one of Berne's two books on groups published in 1963 (the other is PRINCIPLES OF GROUP TREATMENT). This contains a review of the major psychoanalytic group theories and an exposition of Berne's original approach (which is distinct from his theories of transactional analysis). See GROUP APPARATUS, GROUP IMAGO, GROUPS, STAGES OF DEVELOPMENT.

theoretical stance of transactional analysis transactional analysis combines the psychodynamic and developmental viewpoints of psychoanalysis with a concern about the interpersonal context in which the individual operates. The structural theory of ego-states provides an intrapsychic model. The theory of transactions provides an interpersonal one. The theory of functional ego-states (to give one example) links the two by providing a systematic way of relating behaviours to internal states. The result is a model of the individual in a social context that can take account of the dynamics of the whole system. A change in an individual will result in changed behaviours, which will elicit changed behaviours from others and these will impact on the individual. Through their ability to model the whole interpersonal system the theories of transactional analysis are able to offer options for intervention at many points within it.

therapeutic alliance (also called the working alliance) the relationship between therapist and client, which serves to maximise the effectiveness of the therapeutic process. The therapeutic alliance comprises the three domains of bonds, goals and tasks. In transactional analysis the 'OK:OK' position and the contractual process are key aspects of the therapeutic alliance. See also EMPATHY, INTERSUBJECTIVITY.

therapeutic operations Eric Berne (1966) identified a number of operations that play an important role in the therapy process. Most of the operations he described serve mainly to effect DECONTAMINATION of Adult ego-state, two: interpretation and crystallisation, go beyond this into deconfusing the Child ego-state.

Operations mainly effecting decontamination:

1. *Interrogation* (asking questions). Berne advises that this is best used when the client is responding from Adult. Their Child and Parent may block or manipulate, however, it can be used to check on Child beliefs or Parent prejudices. (Asking more questions than are really needed results in playing Psychiatric History.)
2. *Specification* (restating what the client has said to make it clear and/or add more information). This fixes things in the client's mind that can be referred to later.

3. *Confrontation*. This involves using information previously obtained to cross-transact and point out inconsistencies. This stirs up the client and causes a redistribution of cathexis between ego-states. However, this redistribution may reinforce the inappropriate ego-state that is in command if the confrontation is badly timed or badly worded. In Berne's words: 'The therapeutic object is always to cathect the uncontaminated segment of the patient's Adult and its attainment will be signalled by a thoughtful silence or an insightful laugh.'

4. *Explanation*. The therapist says what he or she thinks is going on. This aims to strengthen, decontaminate or reorient the client's Adult.

5. *Illustration*. The therapist tells a story to make a point. Illustration is significantly different to the other interventions. The therapist is *interposing* something between the client's Adult and his or her other ego-states in order to stabilise the Adult and make it more difficult for him or her to slide back into Child or Parent. Berne classified the other therapeutic operations as *interventions* but illustration he describes as an *interposition*.

6. *Confirmation*. The therapist reinforces a point that emerged earlier as the client offers more information. Confirmation may be heard by the client's Parent as confirmation that the Child cannot be trusted. If so the Child will feel trapped by the therapist. Confirmation is strengthening to the Adult because of its logical force and reassuring to the Child because it demonstrates the therapist's strength and alertness.

The next two interventions go beyond decontamination into deconfusing the Child.

7. *Interpretation*. This is an attempt to deconfuse the client's Child by decoding, detoxifying, correcting distortions and regrouping past experiences. Berne advised to go easy on interpretation, which may be intellectualisation rather than thinking.

8. *Crystallisation*. A statement of the client's position from the Adult of the therapist to the Adult of the client so that the client's Adult can make a decision to change. Berne advises not to confuse a Child resolution (which will be broken) with an Adult decision (which will be kept). He recommends that this intervention should not be used until Adult, Child and Parent are prepared.

therapy literally any form of treatment. Often used for psychotherapy or counselling.

therapy contract see TREATMENT CONTRACT.

there and then an emphatic way of referring to the past and not the present (here and now). An understanding of the client's past is of great value in understanding his or her present problems but a preoccupation with the past is often used as a defence against dealing with current life issues. If the therapist joins in this process it constitutes the GAME of Archeology. In psychoanalysis this is referred to as the FLIGHT INTO HISTORY.

thinking cognitive processes that may involve unvoiced speech, the manipulation of images, or abstract ideas. One of Paul Ware's three DOORS TO THERAPY. Cognitive-behavioural and psychodynamic theory give thinking a key position in therapy whereas humanistic approaches stress feeling. Transactional analysis, because of its mixed origins, stands between these positions. Classical transactional analysis (e.g. the writings of Berne) is closer to the psychodynamic view and often more cognitive in its approach than later developments in theory.

thinking disorder the CATHEXIS SCHOOL uses this term to describe certain thinking patterns that are indicative of DISCOUNTING. Two such patterns are *overdetailing,* in which the meaning is lost in a mass of irrelevant detail, and *overgeneralisation,* in which statements are of extreme generality and do not address specific issues.

third force psychology humanistic psychology. The other two 'forces' are psychoanalysis (the psychodynamic approach) and behaviourism. Transactional analysis is a synthesis of all three.

third rule of communication Berne's third rule of communication states that 'the behavioural outcome of an ULTERIOR TRANSACTION is determined at the psychological and not at the social level'. An ulterior transaction operates at two levels. There is a social transaction, which is the ostensible meaning of the transaction and is usually the literal meaning of the words spoken. This meaning is socially acceptable. There is also a second meaning that is understood by both participants. This understanding may not be fully in awareness and certainly will not be acknowledged. This is the psychological level transaction whose content is often not socially acceptable.

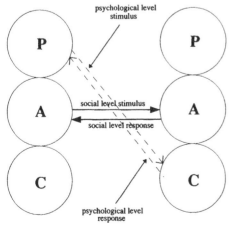

Figure 29 An ulterior transaction (duplex).

three-cornered contract see CONTRACT, THREE-CORNERED.

three Ps Pat Crossman received the Eric Berne Memorial Scientific Award in 1976 for her work on PERMISSION, PROTECTION and POTENCY (Crossman, 1966). These three important concepts are often referred to as 'the three Ps'. The therapist must be able to give the client *permissions* to counteract negative SCRIPT messages such as INJUNCTIONS.

In order to do this they must be perceived by the client as having the *potency* to take on the Parent by being more powerful than the original parent who gave the script messages.

The client's Child ego-state will fear that disastrous consequences may result from disobeying Parental commands and will look to the therapist to provide *protection* against this.

time structuring Berne (1964) suggested that people have a basic need for structure, which he called *structure hunger.* This leads to the development of patterns of time structuring. He identified six such patterns:

withdrawal
rituals
pastimes
(activities)
games
intimacy

Activities differ from the other forms of time structuring in that they are concerned with achieving here-and-now goals. The pursuit of these goals may have a big effect on the process, so the stroke yield and social risk are variable. For the other five patterns stroke yield and social risk tend to rise in the order in which they are listed as involvement and unpredictability rise. For further details see individual entries (WITHDRAWAL etc.).

touching physical contact. There are a wide variety of viewpoints about the use of touching in psychotherapy. Some approaches use it extensively (e.g. Neo-Reichian body work) whereas others forbid it entirely (psychoanalysis). Berne trained as a psychoanalyst and his initial attitude was to minimise touching (even shaking hands, which he did not do until he felt he knew the client). Humanistic influences have shifted attitudes in the direction of using contact more freely, while always noting carefully its significance within the current therapeutic relationship and in the light of what is known of the client's history. Contact that is highly supportive to one client my seem threatening and invasive to another (or even to the same client at a different time) c.f. PRIMAL WOUNDS. Transactional analysis does not have a firm position on this issue and there are wide variations in practice. However there is general agreement among transactional analysts that physical contact is a very significant issue therapeutically and this significance attaches both to the withholding and the giving of contact. However, transactional analysis is a contractual process so any use of touch must be agreed between client and therapist.

tracking the careful following of the client's process, moment by moment, by the therapist or counsellor using intent listening, careful observation and an empathic understanding illuminated by a grasp of relevant theory.

trading stamps see STAMPS.

Training Endorsement Workshop (TEW) a workshop in which certified transactional analysts are trained and endorsed to commence work as trainers of transactional analysis. Those who are successful and go on to train further with a training and supervising transactional analyst (TSTA) have the title 'provisional teaching and supervising transactional analyst' (PTSTA). A

PTSTA can provide officially recognised transactional analysis training and supervision (provided he or she is supervised by a TSTA).

transactional analysis Eric Berne (1961) defined transactional analysis as '. . . a systematic consistent theory of personality and social dynamics derived from clinical experience and an actionistic, rational form of therapy which is suitable for, easily understood by, and naturally adapted to the great majority of psychiatric patients'.

Since Berne wrote this, transactional analysis has found many applications outside of hospital psychotherapy but the elements of his definition – an approach which is rooted in experience, and seeks to be both rational and accessible and points towards clear courses of action – continue to be relevant in all the diverse applications of transactional analysis.

transactional analysis, applications of transactional analysis was originally developed by Eric Berne, a psychiatrist, to work with his patients. The success of *Games People Play* brought his work to the attention of a wide public. Its clarity, accessibility and relevance to a wide spectrum of human behaviour led to its being enthusiastically adopted in many fields other than mental health. It is now used in education, management, staff training and indeed wherever people need to deal with people. Some people also study transactional analysis to develop insight and achieve personal development.

Transactional Analysis in Psychotherapy Berne's major work on transactional analysis, published in 1961. Here is a clear, detailed and comprehensive exposition of his theories. None of his other works deals with the theories of transactional analysis so thoroughly. The style is demanding and clearly directed at the professional, but lightened by Berne's lucid, vivid and at times humorous style. Regrettably, transactional analysis has become best known through Berne's other writings, none of which contains such a comprehensive treatment of transactional analysis theory.

transactional analysis, history of see HISTORY OF TRANSACTIONAL ANALYSIS.

transactional analysis, literature of see LITERATURE OF TRANSACTIONAL ANALYSIS.

transactional analysis, methodology of see METHODOLOGY OF TRANSACTIONAL ANALYSIS.

transactional analysis, philosophy of see PHILOSOPHY OF TRANSACTIONAL ANALYSIS.

transactional analysis proper the analysis of transactions, i.e. determining which ego-states are involved and the type of transaction. The transaction is the point where behaviour and intrapsychic process meet and so is central to transactional analysis, which takes an integrative position involving both viewpoints. This led to the choice of the name of this specific process of analysing transactions for the whole approach.

transactional analysis, schools of see SCHOOLS OF TRANSACTIONAL ANALYSIS.

transactional analysis, special fields see SPECIAL FIELDS.

transactional analysis, theoretical stance see THEORETICAL STANCE OF TRANSACTIONAL ANALYSIS.

transactional response the response that results from a transaction (e.g. what the other person says back).

transactional stimulus an initiating transaction (e.g. saying something to someone else). This is usually followed by a TRANSACTIONAL RESPONSE.

transaction a transaction consists of a transactional stimulus from one person to another (e.g. the first person asks a question) followed by a transactional response (e.g. the second person replies). Berne (1961) described the transaction as the unit of social intercourse.

transactions, analysis of this is referred to as TRANSACTIONAL ANALYSIS PROPER to distinguish it from the therapeutic approach called transactional analysis.

transactions, angular an ulterior transaction in which the psychological level transaction as well as the social level transaction originates from Adult. See also THIRD RULE OF COMMUNICATION, DUPLEX TRANSACTION.

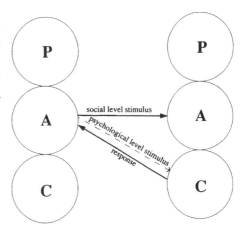

Figure 30 An ulterior transaction (angular).

Salesman to client 'This is the top of the range' (A↔A) 'but it is probably beyond your budget' (A ↔C).

transactions, blocking avoiding discussion of an issue by challenging the definition of the issue c.f. TANGENTIAL TRANSACTIONS.

transactions, complementary a transaction in which the vectors run parallel, indicating consensus about who should be in which ego-state. See FIRST RULE OF COMMUNICATION.

transactions, crossed a transaction in which the vectors are not parallel and in most cases cross. The response is not from the ego-state that was addressed and is not directed to the ego-state that originated the stimulus. See SECOND RULE OF COMMUNICATION.

transactions, duplex the type of ULTERIOR transaction in which the psychological and social level messages pass between different ego-states. See THIRD RULE OF COMMUNICATION, ANGULAR TRANSACTION.

transactions, empathic see EMPATHIC TRANSACTIONS.

transactions, parallel a COMPLEMENTARY transaction.

transaction, tangential a TRANSACTION in which the response is not congruent with the stimulus but addresses a different issue. For example, if the stimulus is a question then the response is an answer to a different question.

transactions, ulterior a transaction in which there are two messages being passed simultaneously, one at the overt or social level and another at the covert or psychological level. See TRANSACTIONS, ANGULAR, TRANSACTIONS, DUPLEX, THIRD RULE OF COMMUNICATION.

transcript an accurate written record of spoken words. Transcripts of psychotherapy sessions are used in the training of transactional analysts to analyse the processes occurring in therapy. The use of such material needs to be agreed in the confidentiality CONTRACT made between therapist or counsellor and his or her client.

transference unawarely transferring attitudes, beliefs and feelings relating to a significant person in the past on to a person in the present such as a therapist. This is sometimes referred to as 'putting a face' on to them. More generally transferring feelings, attitudes and beliefs relevant to some situation in the past on to an analogous situation in the present. This psychoanalytic term was little used in classical transactional analysis, although it is implicit in many transactional analysis concepts. A person in his or her Child or Parent ego-states is not perceiving the world as it now is and so is in transference. Rubberbanding vividly describes what transference feels like from the inside and symbiosis represents a couple bound together in a mutually transferential relationship as seen from the viewpoint of an external observer. Driver behaviour is transferential and discounting is often indicative of transference. The underlying mechanisms of games and script clearly involve transference. In effect transactional analysis tended to substitute operational definitions of how transference manifests itself for the term itself. This suited the behavioural emphasis of transactional analysis in the 1960s and 1970s but was a loss to theory. Modern transactional analysis theorists (e.g. Novellino, 1984, Moiso, 1985) have written extensively on the theory of transference while retaining their rich and unique vocabulary for describing how transference is acted out in behaviour. Clarkson (1992) has developed a classification of types of transference and COUNTERTRANSFERENCE and offers an integrative overview of the use of the concept in modern transactional analysis.

transformational object term used by the psychoanalyst Christopher Bollas (1987). He suggests that the baby's first experience of its mother is of someone or something (perhaps not yet conceived as a person) that transforms self-experience (e.g. by giving comfort). This knowing is more existential than representational. The mother is experienced as a process rather than known as a person. There are parallels in the process of therapy in which the therapist also may transform the client's self-experience. The term may be generalised to any object, person or event that is sought out and used as a transformer of self-experience.

transitional object a concept used by the object relations theorist Donald Winnicott (1951). An object such as a doll, teddy bear or piece of cloth that a child treasures and uses as a comforter. This seems to function as a link between the child and another person (usually the mother) and helps the child to make the transition from dependency to a more independent position.

trauma a damaging experience or set of experiences, particularly as the cause of psychological problems.

treatment contract the agreements made between the therapist or counsellor and his or her client concerning the details of treatment. Transactional analysis is a contractual technique. This means that everything that takes place is agreed. It does not necessarily mean that it is agreed a long time in advance. There will be an overall contract that will specify outcomes. This may be quite general at first, becoming clearer as the work proceeds. There will also be a contracting process in each session to decide a session contract and within the process of the session the therapist will make checks on the client's agreement. See CONTRACT.

treatment planning the process of planning a treatment direction in psychotherapy or counselling. In doing this it is necessary to take account of the CONTRACT and the DIAGNOSIS.

troll Parent another name for the negative aspect of the Parent in Child (P_1). This is also referred to as the witch Parent, the pig Parent, ogre Parent or the electrode.

Try Hard one of the five DRIVERS. When in Try Hard, the person is in SCRIPT, seeking approval from the internal Parent or some person on whom the Parent has been projected. This approval is for effort rather than achievement so people in Try Hard tend to do things the hard way and often fail.

TSTA teaching and supervising transactional analyst. A transactional analyst who is qualified to train and supervise provisional teaching and supervising transactional analysts (PTSTA).

Tuckman's stages of group development see GROUPS, STAGES OF DEVELOPMENT.

two-chair work the client is invited to imagine another person (or sometimes a part of himself or herself) in another chair and to talk to this person. The client may also sit in the other chair and speak as the other person. This enables something that is internal, such as a conception of a significant person (INTROJECT), to be externalised and dealt with by a process of PROJECTION. This technique derives from GESTALT THERAPY. It is extensively used in transactional analysis, often as part of redecision therapy. See REDECISION SCHOOL.

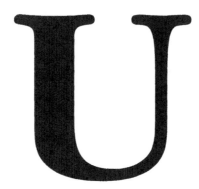

U

UKCP (United Kingdom Council for Psychotherapy) the major governing body for psychotherapy in the UK, which operates a voluntary system of registration for psychotherapists. Training bodies are assessed by a process of peer review and if they reach the standards laid down by the UKCP they are granted full membership. Trainees of member organisations are placed on the register when they qualify. The UK transactional analysis organisation, the Institute of Transactional Analysis, is a full member of UKCP. As a result clinical certified transactional analysts become UKCP registered psychotherapists.

ulterior transaction sometimes shortened to 'ulterior'. A transaction that occurs at two levels: a social level, conveying a message that is socially acceptable, and also at an unspoken psychological level. The psychological level message is usually manipulative or sexual and involves Parent ↔ Child, Child ↔ Child or Parent ↔ Parent transactions whereas the social level message is ostensibly Adult ↔ Adult.

Berne's third rule of communication states that *the behavioural outcome of an ulterior transaction is determined at the psychological and not at the social level.*

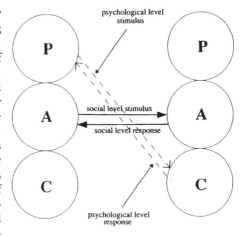

Figure 31 An ulterior transaction (duplex).

unbound energy in Berne's energy theory (Berne, 1961), that part of the psychological energy (CATHEXIS) associated with an ego-state that is available for use. Some energy may remain bound and therefore not available. There is also energy that is free to move between ego-states and is therefore available to cathect any of the ego-states. This is known as *free energy* (or free cathexis). See ENERGY.

unconditional positive regard (Rogerian person-centred therapy) an unconditional acceptance of the intrinsic worth of the other person reflected in a positive attitude towards them. This does not mean unconditional acceptance of their behaviour. This concept is similar to I'M OK, YOU'RE OK and the client-centred approach has been an influence on the way many transactional analysts practise.

unconditioned reflex (behaviourism) a reflex (automatic response) that is not the result of conditioning (training), such as salivating at the sight of food.

unconscious (psychoanalysis) in classical Freudian theory, a zone of the mind whose content is usually inaccessible. Elements of the ego and superego may be unconscious but the major content of the unconscious is instinctual energy associated with the ID as well as disturbing material repressed from the conscious mind. It has no sense of time or consistency (PRIMARY PROCESS THINKING). The term has been little used in transactional analysis although certain concepts (injunctions, the psychological messages of ulterior transactions etc.) might be seen as referring to unconscious structures. Instead, a distinction is often made between what is *in awareness* or *out of awareness*. This classifies the availability of the mental material without making assumptions about the structure of the mind.

unfinished business unresolved issues from the past that are at the root of current emotional or behavioural difficulties. This term, originating in GESTALT, is often used in transactional analysis.

unhappiness a generalised feeling of psychological discomfort that may involve a mixture of emotions and experiences. These may include sadness but unhappiness is not to be equated with sadness, which is one of the FOUR AUTHENTIC FEELINGS. Unhappiness can be a consequence of real sources of distress but it may also be a RACKET FEELING.

United Kingdom Council for Psychotherapy see UKCP.

unipolar affective disorder an emotional disorder characterised by a stable emotional state, which is usually depression. This contrasts with bipolar emotional disorder (often referred to as manic depressive illness) in which there are wide mood swings between depression and elation (hypomania or mania). Cyclothymia is a condition marked by less severe swings of mood. These are the classifications of affective disorders used in the DSM-IV (a diagnostic system often used in the certified transactional analyst examination). See also DEPRESSION.

unthought known a spontaneous manifestation of a past being-state possibly as a mood (Bollas, 1987). In transactional analysis terms this describes one of the ways the Child ego-state may be experienced. See also EXPERIENTIAL MEMORY.

Until script a process script pattern characterised by a tendency to defer actions (in particular actions that yield satisfaction) until some task has been performed e.g. not watching television until the dishes have been washed. People with the Until script have Be Perfect as a principal DRIVER and consequently often have the obsessive compulsive (workaholic) PERSONALITY ADAPTATION.

Uproar a GAME in which a conflict is staged to avoid needing to deal with feelings that are perceived as unacceptable. Berne saw the origins of the game as oedipal.

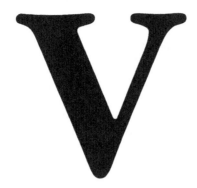

values of transactional analysis see PHI-LOSOPHY OF TRANSACTIONAL ANALYSIS.

vector the line ending in an arrow on a transaction diagram showing the direction of the transaction from the transactional stimulus and the transactional response.

Victim one of the three positions or roles on the DRAMA TRIANGLE. Like the other two positions the Victim position is unauthentic and involves DISCOUNTING.

In this case it is discounting of their power to deal with their own problems. When used in this way the word is spelled with a capital. The Victim role must be distinguished from a real victim who is in real need of help.

violence one of the FOUR PASSIVE BEHAVIOURS.

visualisation generating a picture in the mind. See GUIDED FANTASY, OUTCOME FANTASY.

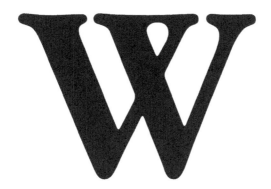

Ware Sequence SEE PERSONALITY ADAPTATION.

warm fuzzies the symbol used for unconditional positive STROKES by CLAUDE STEINER (1974) in his Warm Fuzzy Tale, a children's story that expresses the essentials of his ideas about the STROKE ECONOMY.

What Do You Say After You Say Hello? (1972) Eric Berne's last book published posthumously from manuscripts that were edited after his death. Had he lived to edit it then it probably would have been crisper, shorter and more consistent. However; it is a rich source of his later thinking about transactional analysis and particularly on SCRIPT.

witch Parent one of the names for the negative aspect of the Parent in Child P₁. Also called the pig Parent, the troll Parent and the electrode.

withdrawal one of the six ways of TIME STRUCTURING identified by Eric Berne (1964). Withdrawal involves making no contact with others while perhaps fantasising about doing so.

Wooden Leg a GAME initiated from Victim in which a supposed disability is used to avoid taking responsibility for action. 'How could you expect a person with a wooden leg to dance the jig?'

Workaholic Vann Joines' alternative name for the obsessive-compulsive PERSONALITY ADAPTATION.

working agreement an agreement between therapist and client about how to proceed in therapy (Woollams and Brown, 1978). Transactional analysis is a contractual process – everything that is done is openly agreed. Working agreements form an important part of the ongoing CONTRACTING process.

Why Don't You (Yes But) a GAME in which help (usually advice) is sought but everything that is offered is rejected as unsuitable so that the other party who takes the Rescuer role is invited into Victim. The game which usually pairs with this is I'M ONLY TRYING TO HELP YOU.

133

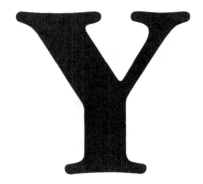

Yes But also known as Why Don't You (Yes But). A GAME in which help (usually advice) is sought but everything that is offered is rejected as unsuitable so that the other party who takes the Rescuer role is invited into Victim. The game that usually pairs with this is I'M ONLY TRYING TO HELP YOU.

You Can't Make Me a GAME initiated from a rebellious Victim position and inviting persecution.

'you' statements 'you' statements often seek to place responsibility for feelings etc. on the other party (for example, 'you made me angry'). Shifting to 'I' statements clarifies the process. 'I feel angry about what you said' owns the feeling and opens up the questions of whether anger is an appropriate response to what has occurred and what is wanted from the other person. 'You' statements are often indicative of Be Strong DRIVER BEHAVIOUR.

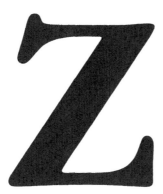

Zalcman, Marilyn transactional analyst. She received the Eric Berne Memorial Scientific Award in 1982 jointly with RICHARD ERSKINE for their work in developing the RACKET SYSTEM (Erskine and Zalcman, 1979). She now conducts training in the US and Europe. For her later thinking on the racket system and racket analysis see Zalcman (1990).

Appendix 1: Reading list

Much of the important literature of transactional analysis is in the *Transactional Analysis Journal* (*TAJ*) which was first published in January 1971. This was preceded by the *Transactional Analysis Bulletin* (*TAB*).

Starting

The TA literature covers a wide range but, because it is a central principle of TA to maximise accessibility, most of it can be attempted once a basic understanding of theory has been obtained. For those with a knowledge of psychology or counselling Berne's *Transactional Analysis in Psychotherapy* (1961) is a good stating point. It is demanding but lucid and contains the most complete exposition of transactional analysis theory in the literature. For those with less background in the field, *Born to Win* by Muriel James and Dorothy Jongeward (1971) is easy to read. *TA Today* by Ian Stewart and Vann Joines (1987) is a recent addition to the literature which is accessible to the beginner but develops theory up to intermediate level. Ian Stewart's *Transactional Analysis Counselling in Action* (Stewart, 1989) offers a clear and accessible introduction to the use of transactional analysis in counselling and his *Eric Berne* (Stewart, 1992) provides an excellent historical and theoretical overview of transactional analysis.

Books by Eric Berne

A Layman's Guide to Psychiatry and Psychoanalysis (originally published 1947 under the title The Mind in Action but extensively revised). This is an early work. The later revised editions (1957, 1967) contain some transactional analysis.

Transactional Analysis in Psychotherapy (1961). Major work.

The Structure and Dynamics of Organizations and Groups (1963). Contains little transactional analysis although it is an important contribution to group theory.

Games People Play (1964). Contains important ideas but games theory has dated.

Principles of Group Treatment (1966). Major work.

Sex in Human Loving (1970). Sex in human relationships in transactional analysis terms.

What Do You Say After You Say Hello? (1972). Berne's last book containing important ideas, particularly about script theory. It has Berne's characteristic, accessible style and is aimed at both a popular and a professional audience. It was edited after his death and would have been crisper and briefer had he lived.

Intuition and Ego States (1977). A compilation of Berne's professional papers published between 1949 and 1962 as he developed transactional analysis.

Some other works illustrating differing approaches

Changing Lives Through Redecision Therapy (1979) Mary and Robert Goulding (a major work of the redecision school).

The Cathexis Reader (1975) Jacqui Lee Schiff et al. A major work of the cathexis school.

Techniques in Transactional Analysis (1977) Edited by Muriel James. Muriel James is both editor and contributing author. Contains a collection of papers on diverse applications of transactional analysis.

Scripts People Live (1974). Claude Steiner (classical school).

Transactional Analysis (1978). Stan Woollams and Michael Brown. A good overview of theory at intermediate level.

Integrative Psychotherapy in Action (1988). Richard Erskine and Janet Moursand. Erskine's integrative approach to transactional analysis.

TA The State of the Art (1984). Edited by Erika Stern. A collection of intermediate to advanced papers originating in Europe.

Transactional Analysis Psychotherapy, An Integrated Approach (1992). Petruska Clarkson. An advanced and comprehensive text from an integrative standpoint.

Transactional Analysis for Trainers (1992). Julie Hay. Transactional analysis from the viewpoint of the organisational special field.

Appendix 2:
Winners of the Eric Berne
Memorial Award

The Eric Berne Memorial Scientific Award was established in 1971 to honour and perpetuate the memory of Eric Berne's scientific contributions. It was to be given annually to the originator of a new scientific concept in transactional analysis.

In 1990, the ITAA Board of Trustees decided to change the title and scope of the Award. It is now known as the Eric Berne Memorial Award in Transactional Analysis. The Award is given annually for published contributions to transactional analysis theory or practice, or for the integration or comparison of transactional analysis theory or practice with other therapeutic modalities. The winner(s) of the Award is (are) chosen by a committee appointed by the ITAA Board of Trustees.

A chronological list of winners of the Award for the years 1971–95 follows, together with references to the works for which they received their awards.

1971
Claude Steiner, SCRIPT MATRIX. Steiner, C. (1966) Script and counterscript. *Transactional Analysis Bulletin* 5(18), 133–5.

1972
Steven Karpman, DRAMA TRIANGLE. Karpman, S. (1968) Fairy tales and script drama analysis. *Transactional Analysis Bulletin* 7(26), 39–43.

1973
John Dusay, EGOGRAMS. Dusay, J. (1972) Egograms and the constancy hypothesis. *Transactional Analysis Journal* 2(3), 137–42.

1974
Aaron Schiff and Jacqui Schiff, PASSIVITY AND THE FOUR DISCOUNTS. Schiff, A. and Schiff, J. (1971) Passivity. *Transactional Analysis Journal* 1(1), 71–8.

1975
Robert Goulding and Mary Goulding, REDECISION AND TWELVE INJUNCTIONS. Goulding, R. and Goulding, M. (1972) New directions in transactional analysis. In Sager and Kaplan (eds) *Progress in Group and Family Therapy*, pp. 105–34. New York: Brunner/Mazel; and (1976) Injunctions, decisions and redecisions. *Transactional Analysis Journal* 6(1), 41–8.

1976
Pat Crossman, PROTECTION. Crossman, P. (1966) Permission and protection. *Transactional Analysis Bulletin* 5(19), 152–4.

1977
Taibi Kahler, MINISCRIPT AND FIVE DRIVERS. Kahler, T. (1974) The miniscript. *Transactional Analysis Journal* 4(1), 26–42.

1978
Fanita English, RACKETS AND REAL FEELINGS: THE SUBSTITUTION FACTOR. English, F. (1971) The substitution factor: rackets and real feelings. *Transactional Analysis Journal* 1(4), 225–30; and (1972) Rackets and real feelings, Part II. *Transactional Analysis Journal* 2(1), 23–5.

1979
Stephen Karpman, OPTIONS. Karpman, S. (1971) Options. *Transactional Analysis Journal* 1(1), 79–87.

1980 (joint award)
Claude Steiner, THE STROKE ECONOMY. Steiner, C. (1971) The stroke economy. *Transactional Analysis Journal* 1(3), 9–15.

Ken Mellor and Eric Sigmund, DISCOUNTING AND REDEFINING. Mellor, K. and Sigmund, E. (1975) Discounting. *Transactional Analysis Journal* 5(3), 295–302; and Mellor, K. and Sigmund, E. (1975) Redefining. *Transactional Analysis Journal* 5(3), 303–11.

1981
Franklin H. Ernst, Jr., THE OK CORRAL. Ernst, F. (1971) The OK corral: the grid for get-on-with. *Transactional Analysis Journal* 1(4), 231–40.

1982
Richard Erskine and Marilyn Zalcman, RACKET SYSTEM AND RACKET ANALYSIS. Erskine, R. and Zalcman, M. (1979) The racket system: a model for racket analysis. *Transactional Analysis Journal* 9(1), 51–9.

1983
Muriel James, SELF-REPARENTING. James, M. (1974) Self-reparenting: theory and process. *Transactional Analysis Journal* 4(3), 32–9.

1984
Pam Levin, DEVELOPMENT CYCLE. Levin, P. (1982) The cycle of development. *Transactional Analysis Journal* 12(2), 129–39.

1985, 1986
Not awarded.

1987
Carlo Moiso, EGO STATES AND TRANSFERENCE. Moiso, C. (1985) Ego states and transference. *Transactional Analysis Journal* 15(3), 194–201.

1988 to 1993
Not awarded.

1994 (EBMA joint award)

Sharon R. Dashiell (area: practice applications). Dashiell, S. (1978) The Parent resolution process: reprogramming psychic incorporations in the parent. *Transactional Analysis Journal* 8(4), 289–94.

John R. McNeel (area: practice applications). McNeel, J. (1976) The Parent interview. *Transactional Analysis Journal* 6(1), 61–8.

Vann S. Joines (area: integration of TA with other theories and approaches). Joines, V. (1986) Using Redecision therapy with different personality adaptations. *Transactional Analysis Journal* 16(3), 152–60; and (1988) Diagnosis and treatment planning using a transactional analysis framework. *Transactional Analysis Journal* 18(3), 185–90.

1995 (EBMA joint award)

Peg Blackstone (area: integration of TA with other theories and approaches). Blackstone, P. (1993) The dynamic Child: integration of second-order structure, object relations, and self psychology. *Transactional Analysis Journal* 23(4), 216–34.

Jean Illsley Clarke (area: practice applications). Illsley Clarke, J. (1981) *Self-Esteem: a Family Affair.* London: HarperCollins.

Alan Jacobs (area: theory). Articles cited include Jacobs, A. (1987) Autocratic power. *Transactional Analysis Journal* 17(3), 59–71.

Appendix 3:
Codes of ethics

Appendix 3 contains the codes of ethics of the Institute of Transactional Analysis (ITA), the European Association for Transactional Analysis (EATA) and the International Association for Transactional Analysis (ITAA).

ITA statement of ethics

This code of ethics is a live document which is constantly under review. The version reproduced here is that current in June 1997.

Recognising that professional ethics are a series of guidelines to what is considered right and wrong, the ITA's Statement of Ethics seeks to promote, in addition, the development of Adult processing in the field of ethics with particular emphasis on establishing a clear Adult contract.

As members of the ITA we accept the principles and philosophy of TA, furthermore we recognise that through our training, certification process and the public listing of practitioners, the ITA promotes the ethical premises and principles in this document and that, where appropriate, members also conform to the ethical principles of external governing bodies such as the United Kingdom Council for Psychotherapy (UKCP).

We also recognise that members may not always utilise these ethical principles and, therefore, that confrontation of a member is sometimes desirable and/or necessary.

We further recognise that should an individual's behaviour show a lack of integration of, or consistency with, these principles, his/her certification, authority to supervise and/or train, training contract and/or membership may be suspended by the ITA until such time as that integration is assured.

These principles represent a consensus of Parent values, Adult data and Child rights:

The term *client* denotes anyone using the services of a member using Transactional Analysis working in any field, and includes individuals, trainees, supervisees, and organisations.

1. An ITA member acknowledges the dignity of all humanity; members of the ITA are expected to conduct themselves in such a way that they promote equal opportunities for all.
2. Members of the ITA shall in their public statements, whether written or verbal, speak with respect and with the intent of furthering professional standing, bearing in mind their responsibility as representatives of the ITA and Transactional Analysis.

142

3. It is the primary protective responsibility of members of the ITA to provide their best possible services to the client and to act in such a way as to cause no avoidable harm to any client.

4. Members of the ITA are committed to develop in their work with clients, an awareness of functioning from a position of dignity, autonomy and personal responsibility.

5. The ethical practice of Transactional Analysis involves entering an informed contractual relationship with the client, which the client as well as the ITA member should have the competence and intent to fulfil. When a client is unable or unwilling to act responsibly within this contractual relationship, the ITA member shall resolve this relationship in such a way as to minimise any harm to the client.

6. A member of the ITA will not exploit a client in any manner, including, but not limited to financial and sexual matters. Sexual relations between an ITA member and a client are prohibited.

7. Members of the ITA will not enter into or maintain a professional contract where other activities or relationships between an ITA member and a client may jeopardise the professional contract.

8. The professional relationship between a member of the ITA and a client is defined by the contract, and that professional relationship ends with the termination of the contract. However certain professional responsibilities continue beyond the termination of the contract. They include but are not limited to the following:

   maintenance of agreed-upon confidentiality
   avoidance of any exploitation of the former relationship
   provision for any needed follow-up care or support

9. Contracts with clients shall be explicit regarding fees, payment schedule, holidays, cancellation of sessions by client or practitioner, and frequency of sessions. The member shall make it clear whether the contract with the client is for therapy, training, supervision, consultancy or some other service. The length of the professional work, the methods utilised, transfers of clients and termination shall be discussed with clients and mutual agreement sought.

10. Members of the ITA will operate and conduct services to clients in compliance with the laws of the country in which they reside and work.

11. In establishing a professional relationship, members of the ITA assume responsibility for providing a suitable environment, including but not limited to such things as specifying the nature and limitations of confidentiality to be observed, providing for physical safety appropriate to the form of activity involved, and obtaining informed consent for any high-risk procedures.

12. If members of the ITA become aware that personal conflicts of medical, financial or other problems might interfere with their ability to carry out a contractual relationship, they must either terminate the contract in a professionally responsible manner, or ensure that the client has the fullest possible information needed to make a decision about remaining in the contractual relationship.

13. Members of the ITA accept responsibility to confront a colleague, whom they have reasonable cause to believe is acting in an unethical manner, and, failing resolution, to report that colleague to the appropriate professional body.

14. In the event that a complaint should be made against a member, that member shall co-operate in resolving such a complaint and will comply in all respects with requirements of the Procedures for Handling Ethics Charges which are current at that time.

15. ITA members who apply Transactional Analysis in their professions will demonstrate a commitment to keep up-to-date in their fields of application through activities such

as further training, conferences and seminars, professional writing and reading, and by being informed of, and promoting the interest of TA.

16. All communication between the member and the client shall be regarded as confidential except as explicitly provided for in the contract or in compliance with relevant law. All members shall maintain records of sessions and these shall be kept confidential in a secure place. Except as agreed in the contract or in compliance with the law, information can be disclosed only with client's consent, unless the practitioner believes that there is convincing evidence of serious danger to the client or others if such information is withheld. Clients must be informed that practitioners may discuss their work with their supervisors. Supervisors and members of a supervision group shall treat material presented with the same care and confidentiality as provided for in the original contract. Particular care will be taken when presenting case material outside of the usual boundaries of supervision, e.g. for training or teaching purposes. In such cases where case material records are present – whether printed, verbal, on tape, firm, or video, or retrieved from electronic media – the client's consent in writing shall be obtained.

EATA code of ethics

A. An EATA member acknowledges the dignity of all humanity.

B. EATA members shall in their public statements refrain from derogatory statements or innuendoes that disparage the standing, qualifications or character of other members, bearing in mind their responsibility as representatives of EATA and Transactional Analysis. On the other hand, direct personal and objective criticism is welcome.

C. It is the primary protective responsibility of EATA members to provide their best possible services to the client and to act in such a way as to cause no harm intentionally or by negligence.

D. EATA members should strive to develop in their clients awareness of and functioning from a position of dignity, autonomy and personal responsibility.

E. The ethical practice of Transactional Analysis involves entering an informed contractual relationship with the client which the client as well as the EATA member should have the competence and intent to fulfil, the EATA member must resolve this relationship in such a way as to bring no harm to the client.

F. An EATA member will not exploit a client in any matter, including, but not limited to financial and sexual matters. Sexual relationships between EATA members and their clients are prohibited.

G. EATA members will not enter into or maintain a professional contract where other activities or relationships between EATA members and clients might jeopardise the professional contract.

H. The professional relationship between an EATA member and the client is defined by the contract. This professional relationship ends with the termination of the contract. However, certain professional responsibilities continue beyond the termination of the contract. They include, but are not limited to, the following:

maintenance of agreed-upon confidentiality
avoidance of any exploitation of the former relationship
provision for any needed follow-up care.

I. EATA members will operate and conduct services to clients with full responsibility to existing laws of the state and/or country in which they reside.

J. In establishing a professional relationship, EATA members assume responsibility for providing a suitable environment for the client, including such things as specifying the nature of confidentiality observed, providing for physical safety appropriate to the form of activity involved and obtaining informed consent for possible high-risk procedures.

K. If EATA members become aware of the fact that personal conflicts or medical problems might interfere with their ability to carry out a contractual relationship, they must either terminate the contract in a professional manner, or ensure that the client has the full information needed to make a decision about remaining in the contractual relationship.

L. EATA members accept responsibility to confront a colleague whom they have reasonable cause to believe is acting in an unethical manner, and, failing resolution, to report that colleague to the appropriate professional body.

M. EATA members who apply Transactional Analysis in their professions will demonstrate a commitment to keep up-to-date in their fields of application through activities such as conferences and seminars, professional writing and reading, as well as to be constantly informed about the TA association's interests.

The ITAA statement of ethics

Recognising that professional ethics are a series of Parent rules as to what is right and wrong the ITAA's Statement of Ethics seeks to promote, in addition, the development of Adult processing in the field of ethics with particular emphasis on establishing a clear Adult contract.

We recognise that through our certification process, the ITAA establishes a social contract that invites the public to trust that Certified Members and Regular Members of the ITAA acknowledge and adhere to the ethical premises and principles in this document.

We also recognise that members do not always utilise these ethical principles and, therefore, that confrontation of a member is sometimes desirable and/or necessary.

We further recognise that should an individual's behaviour show a lack of integration of or consistency with these principles, his/her certification, training contract and/or membership may be suspended by the ITAA until such time as that integration is assured.

These principles represent a consensus of Parent values, Adult data and Child rights:

1. An ITAA member acknowledges the dignity of all humanity regardless of physiological, psychological or economic status.

2. Members of the ITAA shall in their public statements, whether written or verbal, refrain from derogatory statements, inferences and/or innuendoes that disparage the standing, qualifications or character of members, bearing in mind their responsibility as representatives of the ITAA and of transactional analysis.

3. It is the primary protective responsibility of members of the ITAA to provide their best possible services to the client and to act in such a way as to cause no intentional or deliberate harm to any client.

4. Members of the ITAA should strive to develop in their clients awareness of and functioning from a position of dignity, autonomy and personal responsibility.

5. The ethical practice of transactional analysis involves entering into an informed contractual relationship with a client which the member of the ITAA and the client

should have the competence and intent to fulfil. When a client is unable or unwilling to function autonomously and responsibly within this contractual relationship, the member of the ITAA must resolve this relationship in such a way as to bring no harm to the client.

6. A member of the ITAA will not exploit a client in any manner, including, but not limited to, financial and sexual matters. Sexual relations between an ITAA member and a client are prohibited.

7. Members of the ITAA will not enter into or maintain a professional contract where other activities or relationships between an ITAA member and a client might jeopardise the professional contract.

8. The professional relationship between a member of the ITAA and the client is defined by the contract, and that professional relationship ends with the termination of the contract. However, certain professional responsibilities continue beyond the termination of the contract. They include, but are not limited to, the following: a) maintenance of agreed-upon confidentiality; b) avoidance of any exploitation of the former relationship; c) provision for any needed follow-up care.

9. Members of the ITAA will operate and conduct services to clients with full responsibility to existing laws of the state and/or country in which they reside.

10. In establishing a professional relationship, members of the ITAA assume responsibility for providing a suitable environment, including such things as specifying the nature of confidentiality observed, providing for physical safety appropriate to the form of activity involved, and obtaining informed consent for high-risk procedures.

11. If members of the ITAA become aware that personal conflicts or medical problems might interfere with their ability to carry out a contractual relationship, they must either terminate the contract in a professionally responsible manner, or ensure that the client has the full information needed to make a decision about remaining in the contractual relationship.

12. Members of the ITAA accept responsibility to confront a colleague whom they have reasonable cause to believe is acting in an unethical manner, and, failing resolution, to report that colleague to the appropriate professional body.

We affirm these principles as common to the practice of those certified by the ITAA unless a member of ITAA explicitly states in writing his/her differences from these positions. In such an instance, the client's attention to any such differences must also be noted in writing as part of their contract-setting process.

References

TAB Transactional Analysis Bulletin – the ITAA journal before 1971
TAJ Transactional Analysis Journal – the ITAA journal from 1971 onwards
Script a monthly publication of ITAA containing a mix of news and theory articles

Achimovich, L. (1985) Suicidal scripting in the families of anorectics, *TAJ* **15**(1), 21–9.

Bandler, R. and Grinder, J. (1975a) *The Structure of Magic*. Palo Alto: Science and Behaviour Books.

Bandler, R. and Grinder, J. (1975b) *Patterns of the Hypnotic Techniques of Milton Erickson MD*. Cupertino: Meta Publications.

Berne, E. (1947) *The Mind in Action*. New York: Simon & Schuster.

Berne, E. (1957) *A Layman's Guide to Psychiatry and Psychoanalysis*. New York: Simon & Schuster.

Berne, E. (1961) *Transactional Analysis in Psychotherapy*. New York: Grove Press.

Berne, E. (1963) *The Structure and Dynamics of Organizations and Groups*. New York: Grove Press.

Berne, E. (1964) *Games People Play*. New York: Grove Press.

Berne, E. (1966) *Principles of Group Treatment*. New York: Oxford University Press.

Berne, E. (1970) *Sex in Human Loving*. New York: Simon & Schuster.

Berne, E. (1971) Away from a theory of the impact of interpersonal interactions on non-verbal participation. *TAJ* **1**(1), 6–13.

Berne, E. (1972) *What Do You Say After You Say Hello?* New York: Grove Press.

Berne, E. (1977) (ed. P. McCormick) *Intuition and Ego States*. San Francisco: TA Press.

Blackstone, P. (1993) The dynamic child: integration of second-order structure, object relations and self-psychology. *TAJ* **23**, 3.

Bollas, C. (1987) *The Shadow of the Object. The Psychoanalysis of the Unthought Known*. London: Free Association.

Bowlby, J. (1969) *Attachment and Loss*. London: Hogarth and the Institute of Psychoanalysis.

Buber, M. (trans. Kaufman) (1923, 1970) *I and Thou*. Edinburgh: T. & T. Clark.

Cassius, J. (1975) *Body Scripts*. Memphis: Cassius.

Cassius, J. (1977) Bioenergetics and TA. In James, M. (ed) *Techniques in Transactional Analysis*. Reading, MA: Addison-Wesley.

Childs-Gowell, E. and Kinnaman, P. (1978) *Bodyscript Blockbusting: A Transactional Approach to Body Awareness*. San Francisco: Transactional Publications.

Clark, B.D. (1991) Empathic transactions in the deconfusion of Child ego states. *TAJ* **21**(2), 92–8.

Clarke, J.I. (1978) *Self-Esteem, A Family Affair*. Minneapolis: Winston Press.

Clarkson, P. (1987) The bystander role. *TAJ* **17**(3), 82–7.

Clarkson, P. (1992) *Transactional Analysis Psychotherapy, An Integrated Approach*. London: Tavistock/Routledge.

Clarkson, P. (1996) The eclectic and integrative paradigm, between the Scylla of confluence and the Charybdis of confusion. In Woolfe, R. and Dryden, W. *Handbook of Counselling Psychology*. London: Sage. pp 258–84.

Clarkson, P. (1997) *The Bystander (An End to Innocence in Human Relationships?)* London: Whurr.

Clarkson, P. and Fish, S. (1988) Rechilding: creating a new past in the present as a support for the future. *TAJ* **18**(1), 51–9.

Cornell, W. (1994) Shame, binding affect, ego-state contamination and relational repair. *TAJ* **24**(2), 139–46.

Cowles-Boyd, L. (1980) Psychosomatic disturbances and tragic script payoffs. *TAJ* **10**(3), 230–1.

Crossman, P. (1966) Permission and protection. *TAB* **5**(19), 152–4.

Dashiel, S.H. (1978) The Parent resolution process. *TAJ* **10**(4), 289–94.

Dusay, J. (1972) Egograms and the constancy hypothesis. *TAJ* **2**(3), 37–42.

English, F. (1969) Episcript and the 'hot potato' game. *TAB* **8**(32), 77–82.

English, F. (1971) The substitution factor, rackets and real feelings. *TAJ* **1**(4), 225–30.

English, F. (1972) Rackets and real feelings. Part II. *TAJ* **2**(1), 23–5.

English, F. (1975) The three cornered contract. *TAJ* **5**(4), 383–4.

English, F. (1994) Shame and social control revisited. *TAJ* **24**(2), 109–20.

Erikson, E. (1950) *Childhood and Society*. New York: Norton.

Ernst, F.H. (1971) The OK corral: the grid for get-on-with. *TAJ* **1**(4), 231–40.

Erskine, R. (1973) Six stages of treatment. *TAJ* **3**(3), 17–18.

Erskine, R. (1980) Script cure: behavioural, intrapsychic and physiological. *TAJ* **10**(2), 102–6.

Erskine, R. (1993) Inquiry, attunement and involvement in the psychotherapy of dissociation. *TAJ* **23**(4), 184–90.

Erskine, R. (1994) Shame and self-righteousness: transactional analysis perspectives and clinical interventions. *TAJ* **24**(2), 86–102.

Erskine, R. and Moursund, J. (1988) *Integrative Psychotherapy in Action*. Newbury Park, CA: Sage.

Erskine, R. and Trautmann, R. (1993) *The Process of Integrative Psychotherapy*. The Broadwalk Papers: Selections from the 1993 Eastern Regional Transactional Analysis Conference, Atlantic City, N.J. Stamford CT: Eastern Regional Transactional Analysis Association.

Erskine, R.G. and Zalcman, M. (1979) The racket system: a model for racket analysis. *TAJ* **9**(1), 51–9.

Fairbairn, W.R.D. (1952) *Psycho-analytic Studies of the Personality*. London: Tavistock.

Feltham, C. and Dryden, W. (1993) *Dictionary of Counselling*. London: Whurr.

Fukazawa, M. (1977) A child of wealth and growth: a case of anorexia in Japan. *TAJ* **7**(1), 73–6.

Goode, E. (1985) Medical aspects of the bulimic syndrome and bulimarexia, *TAJ* **15**(1), 4–11.

Goulding, R. and Goulding, M. (1972) in Sager and Kaplan (eds) *Progress in Group and Family Therapy*, New York, Brunner/Mazel, pp 105–34.

Goulding, M. and Goulding, R. (1979) *Changing Lives Through Redecision Therapy*. New York: Grove Press.

Goulding, R. and Goulding, M. (1976) Injunction, decisions and redecisions. *TAJ* **6**(1), 41–8.

Grof, Stanislav (1985), *Beyond the Brain: Birth, Death, and Transcendence in Psychotherapy*, Albany, State University of New York Press.

Hay, J. (1992) *Transactional Analysis for Trainers*, London, McGraw-Hill.

Hine, J. (1990) The bilateral and ongoing nature of games. *TAJ* **20**(1), 28–39.

Holloway, W. (1973) *Shut the Escape*

Hatch. Ohio: Midwest Institute of Human Understanding Inc.

International Transactional Analysis Association (1995) *Transactional Analysis Counseling Definition.* San Francisco, CA: Training and Certification Council of Transactional Analysts, Training Standards Committee, Counseling Task Force.

Jacobs, A. (1991) Groups, organizations, nations and players. *TAJ* **21**(4), 199–206.

James, J. (1973) The game plan. *TAJ* **3**(4), 14–17.

James, M. (1974) Self-reparenting: theory and process. *TAJ* **12**(2), 32–9.

James, M. (ed) (1977) *Techniques in Transactional Analysis for Psychotherapists and Counsellors,* Reading, Addison-Wesley.

James, M. and Jongeward, D. (1971) *Born to Win: transactional analysis with Gestalt experiments,* Reading, Addison-Wesley.

Joines, V. (1986) Using redecision therapy with different personality adaptations. *TAJ* **16**(3), 152–60.

Joines, V. (1988) Diagnosis and treatment planning using a transactional analysis framework. *TAJ* **18**(3), 185–90.

Kahler, T. (1978) *Transactional Analysis Revisited.* Little Rock: Human Development Publications.

Kahler, T. and Capers, H. (1974) The miniscript. *TAJ* **4**(1), 26–42.

Karpman, S. (1968) Fairy tales and script drama analysis. *TAB* **7**(26), 39–43.

Karpman, S. (1971) Options. *TAJ* **1**(1), 79–87.

Kubler-Ross, E. (1969) *On Death and Dying.* New York: Macmillan.

Lacousiere, R. (1980) *The Life Cycle of Groups.* New York: Life Sciences Press.

Lee, Adrienne (1988a) Scriptbound – private communication.

Lee, Adrienne (1988b) Primal Wounds – private communication.

Lee, Adrienne (1997) Process contracts. In Sills, S. (ed.) *Contracts in Counselling.* London: Sage.

Levin, P. (1974) *Becoming the Way We Are:* *a transactional analysis guide to personal development,* Berkeley, Levin.

Levin, P. (1982) The cycle of development. *TAJ* **12**(2), 129–39.

Levin, P. (1988) *Cycles of Power.* Deerfield Beach: Health Communications.

Liddell and Scott (1935) *Greek–English Lexicon.* Oxford: Clarendon.

Loomis, M. and Landsman, S. (1980) Manic-depressive structure: assessment and development. *TAJ* **10**(4), 284–90.

Mahler, M. (1975) *The Psychological Birth of the Human Infant.* New York: Basic Books.

Maine, M. (1985) Effective treatment of anorexia nervosa, the recovered patient's view. *TAJ* **15**(1), 48–54.

McDevitt, J. and Mahler, M. (1980) Object constancy, individuality and internalization. In Greenspan, S. and Pollock, G. (eds) *The Course of Life.* Washington DC: US Government Printing Office. pp. 407–24.

McDougall, J. (1989) *Theatres of the Body.* London: Free Association.

McNeel, J. (1976) The Parent interview. *TAJ* **6**(1), 61–8.

Mellor, K. (1980) Impasses: a developmental and structural understanding. *TAJ* **10**(3), 213–21.

Mellor, K. and Andrewartha, G. (1980) Reparenting the Parent in support of redecisions. *TAJ* 10, 3, 197–203.

Mellor, K. and Sigmund, E. (1975a) Discounting. *TAJ* **5**(3), 295–302.

Mellor, K. and Sigmund, E. (1975b) Redefining *TAJ* **5**(3), 303–11.

Merlin, E. (1977) *Analytical Psychology and TA.* In James, M. (ed.) *Techniques in Transactional Analysis.* Reading MA: Addison-Wesley. pp. 217–38.

Miller, A. (1983) *The Drama of the Gifted Child.* London: Faber.

Miller, A. (1985) *Thou Shalt Not Be Aware: Society's Betrayal of The Child.* London: Pluto Books.

Moiso, C. (1984) The feeling loop. In Stern E. (ed.) *TA The State of the Art.* Dordrecht: Foris Publications. pp. 69–76.

Moiso, C. (1985) Ego states and transference. *TAJ* **15**(3), 194–201.

Novellino, M. (1984) Self-analysis of transference in integrative transactional analysis. *TAJ* **14**(1), 63–7.

Novey, T. (1997) Comparing Bernian and Freudian personality models. *Script* **27**(2), 3.

Osnes, R.E. (1974) Spot reparenting. *TAJ* **4**(3), 40–6.

Rogers, C.R. (1951) *Client-centred Therapy, Its Current Practice, Implications and Theory*. Boston: Houghton Mifflin.

Rogers, C.R. (1961) *On Becoming a Person*. Boston: Houghton Mifflin.

Rutter, M. (1972) *Maternal Deprivation Reassessed*. Harmondsworth: Penguin.

Schiff, J.L. and Day, B. (1970) *All My Children*. New York: Pyramid Publications.

Schiff, A.W. and Schiff, J.L. (1971) Passivity. *TAJ* **1**(1), 71–8.

Schiff J.L. et al. (1975) *The Cathexis Reader: Transactional Analysis Treatment of Psychosis*. New York: Harper & Row.

Steere, D. (1982) *Bodily Expression in Psychotherapy*. New York: Brunner/Mazel.

Steiner, C. (1966) Script and counterscript. *TAJ* **5**(18), 133–5.

Steiner, C. (1971) The stroke economy. *TAJ* **1**(3), 9–15.

Steiner, C. (1971) *Games Alcoholics Play*. New York: Grove Press.

Steiner, C. (1974) *Scripts People Live*. New York: Grove Press.

Stern, D. (1985) *The Interpersonal World of the Infant*. New York: Basic Books.

Stewart, I. (1989) *Transactional Analysis Counselling in Action*. London: Sage.

Stewart, I. (1992) *Eric Berne*. London: Sage.

Stewart, I. (1996a) *History of Transactional Analysis*. In Dryden, W. (ed.) *Developments in Psychotherapy, Historical Perspectives*. London: Sage.

Stewart, I. (1996b) *Developing Transactional Analysis Counselling*. London: Sage.

Stewart, I. and Joines, V. (1987) *TA Today*. Nottingham: Lifespace.

Stuntz, E.C. (1973) Multiple chairs technique. *TAJ* **3**(2), 29.

Sullivan, H.S. (1953) *The Interpersonal Theory of Psychiatry*. New York: Norton.

Szasz, T. (1961) *The Myth of Mental Illness: Foundations of a Therapy of Personal Conduct*. New York: Hoeber-Harper.

Tuckman, B.W. (1965) Developmental sequences in small groups. *Psychological Bulletin* **63**(6), 384–99.

Tuckman, B.W. and Jensen, M.A.C. (1977) Stages of small group development. *Journal of Group and Organizational Studies* **2**, 419–27.

Vognsen, J. (1985) Brief strategic treatment of bulimia. *TAJ* **15**(1), 79–84.

Ware, P. (1983) Personality adaptations. *TAJ* **13**(1), 11–19.

Weiss, L. and Weiss, J. (1984) The good child syndrome. In Stern, E. (ed.) *TA, The State of the Art*. Dordrecht, Holland: Foris. pp. 119–26.

Winnicott, D. (1951) Transitional objects and transitional phenomena. Reprinted in (1975) *Collected Papers: Through Paediatrics to Psychoanalysis*. London: Tavistock.

Winnicott, D. (1964) *The Child, the Family and the Outside World*. Harmondsworth: Penguin.

Winnicott, D. (1971) *Playing and Reality*. London: Tavistock.

Woollams, S. and Brown, M. (1978) *Transactional Analysis*. Dexter: Huron Valley Press.

Zalcman, M. (1990), Game Analysis and Racket Analysis: Overview, Critique and Future Developments, *TAJ* **20**, 1, 4–19.

Zalcman, M. and Erskine, R. (1979) The racket system: a model for racket analysis. *TAJ* **9**(1), 51–9.

Zeichnich, R. (1968) Paranoia. *TAB* **7**(26), 44.

Printed and bound by CPI Group (UK) Ltd, Croydon, CR0 4YY

09/06/2025

14686006-0001